GRATITUDE

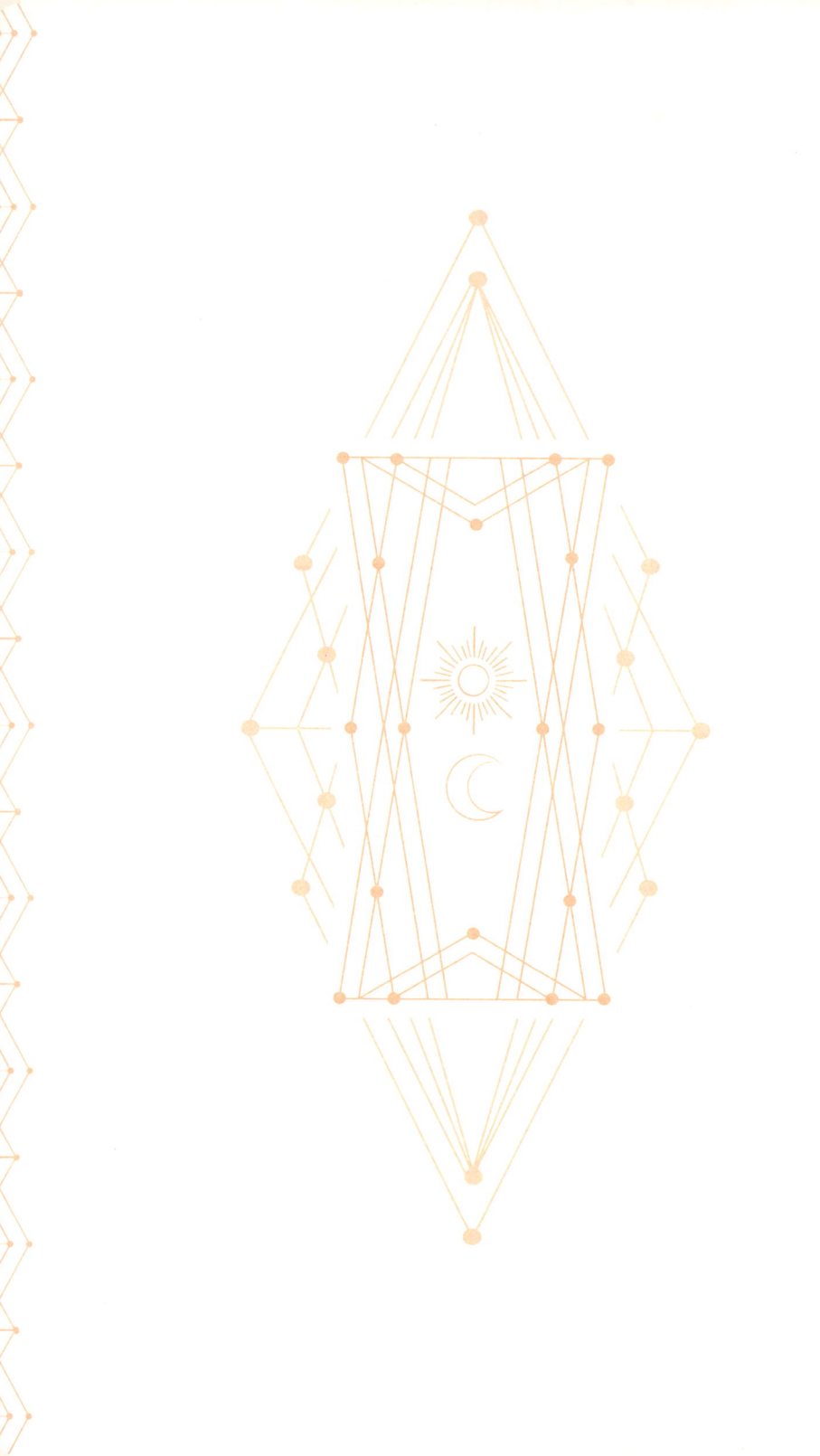

KEEPING A GRATITUDE JOURNAL is an effective way to feel happier and more motivated in your day-to-day life. Regular attention to this journal will encourage you to focus more on things that inspire and enrich you and less on things that drain your energy and resources.

The prompts in this journal will guide you to reflect on the people, things, and events that fill your heart with appreciation and joy. You can record big accomplishments, like running a marathon, and small delights, like your morning cup of tea. What matters most is that you recognize the good emotions associated with writing gratitude entries and notice how they impact your everyday life.

Designed to be annotated twice a day, this journal prompts you to set out with a positive mood each morning and reflect thankfully on the day's events and emotions each evening. Take your time writing entries, savor every new experience, and enjoy the gifts that gratitude can bring to each moment.

MORNING

DATE ___/___/___

TODAY'S FOCUS:
_____
_____
_____
_____

AN AFFIRMATION FOR TODAY:
_____
_____
_____
_____

WHAT I'M GRATEFUL FOR:
_____
_____
_____
_____
_____
_____
_____
_____

WHAT I'M EXCITED ABOUT TODAY:
_____
_____
_____

HOW I'LL MAKE SPACE FOR GRATITUDE TODAY:
_____
_____
_____

EVENING

GOOD THINGS THAT HAPPENED TODAY:
_____
_____
_____
_____

THINGS I DID TO MAKE A POSITIVE DIFFERENCE TODAY:
_____
_____
_____
_____

HOW I FELT TODAY:

- ☐ HAPPY
- ☐ CONTENT
- ☐ PROUD
- ☐ HOPEFUL
- ☐ LOVING
- ☐ CONNECTED
- ☐ BALANCED
- ☐ JOYFUL
- ☐ RELAXED
- ☐ CREATIVE
- ☐ EXCITED
- ☐ _____

- ☐ NEUTRAL
- ☐ INSECURE
- ☐ DISCOURAGED
- ☐ DRAINED
- ☐ SAD
- ☐ SCARED
- ☐ ANGRY
- ☐ ANNOYED
- ☐ ANXIOUS
- ☐ STRESSED
- ☐ OVERWHELMED
- ☐ _____

A POSITIVE THOUGHT TO CARRY ME TO SLEEP:
_____
_____
_____

MORNING

DATE ___/___/___

TODAY'S FOCUS:
___
___
___
___

AN AFFIRMATION FOR TODAY:
___
___
___

WHAT I'M GRATEFUL FOR:
___
___
___
___
___
___
___
___
___

WHAT I'M EXCITED ABOUT TODAY:
___
___
___

HOW I'LL MAKE SPACE FOR GRATITUDE TODAY:
___
___
___

EVENING

GOOD THINGS THAT HAPPENED TODAY:
_____
_____
_____
_____

THINGS I DID TO MAKE A POSITIVE DIFFERENCE TODAY:
_____
_____
_____
_____

HOW I FELT TODAY:

- ☐ HAPPY
- ☐ CONTENT
- ☐ PROUD
- ☐ HOPEFUL
- ☐ LOVING
- ☐ CONNECTED
- ☐ BALANCED
- ☐ JOYFUL
- ☐ RELAXED
- ☐ CREATIVE
- ☐ EXCITED
- ☐ _____

- ☐ NEUTRAL
- ☐ INSECURE
- ☐ DISCOURAGED
- ☐ DRAINED
- ☐ SAD
- ☐ SCARED
- ☐ ANGRY
- ☐ ANNOYED
- ☐ ANXIOUS
- ☐ STRESSED
- ☐ OVERWHELMED
- ☐ _____

_____
_____
_____
_____
_____
_____

A POSITIVE THOUGHT TO CARRY ME TO SLEEP:
_____
_____
_____

MORNING

DATE ___ / ___ / ___

TODAY'S FOCUS:

AN AFFIRMATION FOR TODAY:

WHAT I'M GRATEFUL FOR:

WHAT I'M EXCITED ABOUT TODAY:

HOW I'LL MAKE SPACE FOR GRATITUDE TODAY:

EVENING

GOOD THINGS THAT HAPPENED TODAY:
_____
_____
_____
_____

THINGS I DID TO MAKE A POSITIVE DIFFERENCE TODAY:
_____
_____
_____
_____

HOW I FELT TODAY:

- [ ] HAPPY
- [ ] CONTENT
- [ ] PROUD
- [ ] HOPEFUL
- [ ] LOVING
- [ ] CONNECTED
- [ ] BALANCED
- [ ] JOYFUL
- [ ] RELAXED
- [ ] CREATIVE
- [ ] EXCITED
- [ ] _____

- [ ] NEUTRAL
- [ ] INSECURE
- [ ] DISCOURAGED
- [ ] DRAINED
- [ ] SAD
- [ ] SCARED
- [ ] ANGRY
- [ ] ANNOYED
- [ ] ANXIOUS
- [ ] STRESSED
- [ ] OVERWHELMED
- [ ] _____

_____
_____
_____
_____
_____
_____

A POSITIVE THOUGHT TO CARRY ME TO SLEEP:
_____
_____
_____

MORNING

DATE ___/___/___

TODAY'S FOCUS:
_____
_____
_____
_____

AN AFFIRMATION FOR TODAY:
_____
_____
_____
_____

WHAT I'M GRATEFUL FOR:
_____
_____
_____
_____
_____
_____
_____
_____
_____
_____

WHAT I'M EXCITED ABOUT TODAY:
_____
_____
_____

HOW I'LL MAKE SPACE FOR GRATITUDE TODAY:
_____
_____
_____

EVENING

GOOD THINGS THAT HAPPENED TODAY:
_____
_____
_____
_____

THINGS I DID TO MAKE A POSITIVE DIFFERENCE TODAY:
_____
_____
_____

HOW I FELT TODAY:

- ☐ HAPPY
- ☐ CONTENT
- ☐ PROUD
- ☐ HOPEFUL
- ☐ LOVING
- ☐ CONNECTED
- ☐ BALANCED
- ☐ JOYFUL
- ☐ RELAXED
- ☐ CREATIVE
- ☐ EXCITED
- ☐ _____

- ☐ NEUTRAL
- ☐ INSECURE
- ☐ DISCOURAGED
- ☐ DRAINED
- ☐ SAD
- ☐ SCARED
- ☐ ANGRY
- ☐ ANNOYED
- ☐ ANXIOUS
- ☐ STRESSED
- ☐ OVERWHELMED
- ☐ _____

_____
_____
_____
_____
_____
_____

A POSITIVE THOUGHT TO CARRY ME TO SLEEP:
_____
_____
_____

MORNING

DATE ___/___/___

TODAY'S FOCUS:
_____
_____
_____
_____

AN AFFIRMATION FOR TODAY:
_____
_____
_____
_____

WHAT I'M GRATEFUL FOR:
_____
_____
_____
_____
_____
_____
_____
_____
_____

WHAT I'M EXCITED ABOUT TODAY:
_____
_____
_____

HOW I'LL MAKE SPACE FOR GRATITUDE TODAY:
_____
_____
_____

EVENING

GOOD THINGS THAT HAPPENED TODAY:
_____
_____
_____
_____

THINGS I DID TO MAKE A POSITIVE DIFFERENCE TODAY:
_____
_____
_____

HOW I FELT TODAY:

- ☐ HAPPY
- ☐ CONTENT
- ☐ PROUD
- ☐ HOPEFUL
- ☐ LOVING
- ☐ CONNECTED
- ☐ BALANCED
- ☐ JOYFUL
- ☐ RELAXED
- ☐ CREATIVE
- ☐ EXCITED
- ☐ _____

- ☐ NEUTRAL
- ☐ INSECURE
- ☐ DISCOURAGED
- ☐ DRAINED
- ☐ SAD
- ☐ SCARED
- ☐ ANGRY
- ☐ ANNOYED
- ☐ ANXIOUS
- ☐ STRESSED
- ☐ OVERWHELMED
- ☐ _____

_____
_____
_____
_____
_____
_____

A POSITIVE THOUGHT TO CARRY ME TO SLEEP:
_____
_____
_____

MORNING

DATE ___/___/___

TODAY'S FOCUS:
_____
_____
_____
_____

AN AFFIRMATION FOR TODAY:
_____
_____
_____

WHAT I'M GRATEFUL FOR:
_____
_____
_____
_____
_____
_____
_____
_____
_____

WHAT I'M EXCITED ABOUT TODAY:
_____
_____
_____

HOW I'LL MAKE SPACE FOR GRATITUDE TODAY:
_____
_____
_____

EVENING

GOOD THINGS THAT HAPPENED TODAY:
_____
_____
_____
_____

THINGS I DID TO MAKE A POSITIVE DIFFERENCE TODAY:
_____
_____
_____
_____

HOW I FELT TODAY:

- ☐ HAPPY
- ☐ CONTENT
- ☐ PROUD
- ☐ HOPEFUL
- ☐ LOVING
- ☐ CONNECTED
- ☐ BALANCED
- ☐ JOYFUL
- ☐ RELAXED
- ☐ CREATIVE
- ☐ EXCITED
- ☐ _____

- ☐ NEUTRAL
- ☐ INSECURE
- ☐ DISCOURAGED
- ☐ DRAINED
- ☐ SAD
- ☐ SCARED
- ☐ ANGRY
- ☐ ANNOYED
- ☐ ANXIOUS
- ☐ STRESSED
- ☐ OVERWHELMED
- ☐ _____

A POSITIVE THOUGHT TO CARRY ME TO SLEEP:
_____
_____
_____

MORNING

DATE ___/___/___

TODAY'S FOCUS:
_____
_____
_____
_____

AN AFFIRMATION FOR TODAY:
_____
_____
_____
_____

WHAT I'M GRATEFUL FOR:
_____
_____
_____
_____
_____
_____
_____
_____
_____

WHAT I'M EXCITED ABOUT TODAY:
_____
_____
_____

HOW I'LL MAKE SPACE FOR GRATITUDE TODAY:
_____
_____
_____

EVENING

GOOD THINGS THAT HAPPENED TODAY:
_____
_____
_____
_____

THINGS I DID TO MAKE A POSITIVE DIFFERENCE TODAY:
_____
_____
_____
_____

HOW I FELT TODAY:

- ☐ HAPPY
- ☐ CONTENT
- ☐ PROUD
- ☐ HOPEFUL
- ☐ LOVING
- ☐ CONNECTED
- ☐ BALANCED
- ☐ JOYFUL
- ☐ RELAXED
- ☐ CREATIVE
- ☐ EXCITED
- ☐ _____

- ☐ NEUTRAL
- ☐ INSECURE
- ☐ DISCOURAGED
- ☐ DRAINED
- ☐ SAD
- ☐ SCARED
- ☐ ANGRY
- ☐ ANNOYED
- ☐ ANXIOUS
- ☐ STRESSED
- ☐ OVERWHELMED
- ☐ _____

A POSITIVE THOUGHT TO CARRY ME TO SLEEP:
_____
_____
_____

MORNING

DATE ___/___/___

TODAY'S FOCUS:

AN AFFIRMATION FOR TODAY:

WHAT I'M GRATEFUL FOR:

WHAT I'M EXCITED ABOUT TODAY:

HOW I'LL MAKE SPACE FOR GRATITUDE TODAY:

EVENING

GOOD THINGS THAT HAPPENED TODAY:

_____
_____
_____
_____

THINGS I DID TO MAKE A POSITIVE DIFFERENCE TODAY:

_____
_____
_____
_____

HOW I FELT TODAY:

- ☐ HAPPY
- ☐ CONTENT
- ☐ PROUD
- ☐ HOPEFUL
- ☐ LOVING
- ☐ CONNECTED
- ☐ BALANCED
- ☐ JOYFUL
- ☐ RELAXED
- ☐ CREATIVE
- ☐ EXCITED
- ☐ _____

- ☐ NEUTRAL
- ☐ INSECURE
- ☐ DISCOURAGED
- ☐ DRAINED
- ☐ SAD
- ☐ SCARED
- ☐ ANGRY
- ☐ ANNOYED
- ☐ ANXIOUS
- ☐ STRESSED
- ☐ OVERWHELMED
- ☐ _____

A POSITIVE THOUGHT TO CARRY ME TO SLEEP:

_____
_____
_____

MORNING

DATE ___/___/___

TODAY'S FOCUS:
_____
_____
_____
_____

AN AFFIRMATION FOR TODAY:
_____
_____
_____

WHAT I'M GRATEFUL FOR:
_____
_____
_____
_____
_____
_____
_____
_____
_____

WHAT I'M EXCITED ABOUT TODAY:
_____
_____
_____

HOW I'LL MAKE SPACE FOR GRATITUDE TODAY:
_____
_____
_____

EVENING

GOOD THINGS THAT HAPPENED TODAY:
_____
_____
_____
_____

THINGS I DID TO MAKE A POSITIVE DIFFERENCE TODAY:
_____
_____
_____
_____

HOW I FELT TODAY:

- ☐ HAPPY
- ☐ CONTENT
- ☐ PROUD
- ☐ HOPEFUL
- ☐ LOVING
- ☐ CONNECTED
- ☐ BALANCED
- ☐ JOYFUL
- ☐ RELAXED
- ☐ CREATIVE
- ☐ EXCITED
- ☐ _____

- ☐ NEUTRAL
- ☐ INSECURE
- ☐ DISCOURAGED
- ☐ DRAINED
- ☐ SAD
- ☐ SCARED
- ☐ ANGRY
- ☐ ANNOYED
- ☐ ANXIOUS
- ☐ STRESSED
- ☐ OVERWHELMED
- ☐ _____

A POSITIVE THOUGHT TO CARRY ME TO SLEEP:
_____
_____
_____

MORNING

DATE ___/___/___

TODAY'S FOCUS:
_____
_____
_____
_____

AN AFFIRMATION FOR TODAY:
_____
_____
_____
_____

WHAT I'M GRATEFUL FOR:
_____
_____
_____
_____
_____
_____
_____
_____
_____

WHAT I'M EXCITED ABOUT TODAY:
_____
_____
_____

HOW I'LL MAKE SPACE FOR GRATITUDE TODAY:
_____
_____
_____

EVENING

GOOD THINGS THAT HAPPENED TODAY:
_____
_____
_____
_____

THINGS I DID TO MAKE A POSITIVE DIFFERENCE TODAY:
_____
_____
_____
_____

HOW I FELT TODAY:

- ☐ HAPPY
- ☐ CONTENT
- ☐ PROUD
- ☐ HOPEFUL
- ☐ LOVING
- ☐ CONNECTED
- ☐ BALANCED
- ☐ JOYFUL
- ☐ RELAXED
- ☐ CREATIVE
- ☐ EXCITED
- ☐ _____

- ☐ NEUTRAL
- ☐ INSECURE
- ☐ DISCOURAGED
- ☐ DRAINED
- ☐ SAD
- ☐ SCARED
- ☐ ANGRY
- ☐ ANNOYED
- ☐ ANXIOUS
- ☐ STRESSED
- ☐ OVERWHELMED
- ☐ _____

A POSITIVE THOUGHT TO CARRY ME TO SLEEP:
_____
_____
_____

MORNING

DATE ___ / ___ / ___

TODAY'S FOCUS:

AN AFFIRMATION FOR TODAY:

WHAT I'M GRATEFUL FOR:

WHAT I'M EXCITED ABOUT TODAY:

HOW I'LL MAKE SPACE FOR GRATITUDE TODAY:

EVENING

GOOD THINGS THAT HAPPENED TODAY:
_____
_____
_____
_____

THINGS I DID TO MAKE A POSITIVE DIFFERENCE TODAY:
_____
_____
_____
_____

HOW I FELT TODAY:

- ☐ HAPPY
- ☐ CONTENT
- ☐ PROUD
- ☐ HOPEFUL
- ☐ LOVING
- ☐ CONNECTED
- ☐ BALANCED
- ☐ JOYFUL
- ☐ RELAXED
- ☐ CREATIVE
- ☐ EXCITED
- ☐ _____

- ☐ NEUTRAL
- ☐ INSECURE
- ☐ DISCOURAGED
- ☐ DRAINED
- ☐ SAD
- ☐ SCARED
- ☐ ANGRY
- ☐ ANNOYED
- ☐ ANXIOUS
- ☐ STRESSED
- ☐ OVERWHELMED
- ☐ _____

A POSITIVE THOUGHT TO CARRY ME TO SLEEP:
_____
_____
_____

MORNING

DATE ___/___/___

TODAY'S FOCUS:

AN AFFIRMATION FOR TODAY:

WHAT I'M GRATEFUL FOR:

WHAT I'M EXCITED ABOUT TODAY:

HOW I'LL MAKE SPACE FOR GRATITUDE TODAY:

EVENING

GOOD THINGS THAT HAPPENED TODAY:
_____
_____
_____
_____

THINGS I DID TO MAKE A POSITIVE DIFFERENCE TODAY:
_____
_____
_____
_____

HOW I FELT TODAY:

- ☐ HAPPY
- ☐ CONTENT
- ☐ PROUD
- ☐ HOPEFUL
- ☐ LOVING
- ☐ CONNECTED
- ☐ BALANCED
- ☐ JOYFUL
- ☐ RELAXED
- ☐ CREATIVE
- ☐ EXCITED
- ☐ _____

- ☐ NEUTRAL
- ☐ INSECURE
- ☐ DISCOURAGED
- ☐ DRAINED
- ☐ SAD
- ☐ SCARED
- ☐ ANGRY
- ☐ ANNOYED
- ☐ ANXIOUS
- ☐ STRESSED
- ☐ OVERWHELMED
- ☐ _____

A POSITIVE THOUGHT TO CARRY ME TO SLEEP:
_____
_____
_____

MORNING

DATE ____/____/____

TODAY'S FOCUS:
_____
_____
_____
_____

AN AFFIRMATION FOR TODAY:
_____
_____
_____
_____

WHAT I'M GRATEFUL FOR:
_____
_____
_____
_____
_____
_____
_____
_____
_____

WHAT I'M EXCITED ABOUT TODAY:
_____
_____
_____

HOW I'LL MAKE SPACE FOR GRATITUDE TODAY:
_____
_____
_____

EVENING

GOOD THINGS THAT HAPPENED TODAY:

THINGS I DID TO MAKE A POSITIVE DIFFERENCE TODAY:

HOW I FELT TODAY:

- ☐ HAPPY
- ☐ CONTENT
- ☐ PROUD
- ☐ HOPEFUL
- ☐ LOVING
- ☐ CONNECTED
- ☐ BALANCED
- ☐ JOYFUL
- ☐ RELAXED
- ☐ CREATIVE
- ☐ EXCITED
- ☐ _____

- ☐ NEUTRAL
- ☐ INSECURE
- ☐ DISCOURAGED
- ☐ DRAINED
- ☐ SAD
- ☐ SCARED
- ☐ ANGRY
- ☐ ANNOYED
- ☐ ANXIOUS
- ☐ STRESSED
- ☐ OVERWHELMED
- ☐ _____

A POSITIVE THOUGHT TO CARRY ME TO SLEEP:

MORNING

DATE ___/___/___

TODAY'S FOCUS:
_____
_____
_____
_____

AN AFFIRMATION FOR TODAY:
_____
_____
_____
_____

WHAT I'M GRATEFUL FOR:
_____
_____
_____
_____
_____
_____
_____
_____
_____

WHAT I'M EXCITED ABOUT TODAY:
_____
_____
_____

HOW I'LL MAKE SPACE FOR GRATITUDE TODAY:
_____
_____
_____

EVENING

GOOD THINGS THAT HAPPENED TODAY:
_____
_____
_____

THINGS I DID TO MAKE A POSITIVE DIFFERENCE TODAY:
_____
_____
_____

HOW I FELT TODAY:

- [ ] HAPPY
- [ ] CONTENT
- [ ] PROUD
- [ ] HOPEFUL
- [ ] LOVING
- [ ] CONNECTED
- [ ] BALANCED
- [ ] JOYFUL
- [ ] RELAXED
- [ ] CREATIVE
- [ ] EXCITED
- [ ] _____

- [ ] NEUTRAL
- [ ] INSECURE
- [ ] DISCOURAGED
- [ ] DRAINED
- [ ] SAD
- [ ] SCARED
- [ ] ANGRY
- [ ] ANNOYED
- [ ] ANXIOUS
- [ ] STRESSED
- [ ] OVERWHELMED
- [ ] _____

A POSITIVE THOUGHT TO CARRY ME TO SLEEP:
_____
_____
_____

MORNING

DATE ___/___/___

TODAY'S FOCUS:
_____
_____
_____
_____

AN AFFIRMATION FOR TODAY:
_____
_____
_____
_____

WHAT I'M GRATEFUL FOR:
_____
_____
_____
_____
_____
_____
_____
_____

WHAT I'M EXCITED ABOUT TODAY:
_____
_____
_____

HOW I'LL MAKE SPACE FOR GRATITUDE TODAY:
_____
_____
_____

EVENING

GOOD THINGS THAT HAPPENED TODAY:
_____
_____
_____
_____

THINGS I DID TO MAKE A POSITIVE DIFFERENCE TODAY:
_____
_____
_____
_____

HOW I FELT TODAY:

- [ ] HAPPY
- [ ] CONTENT
- [ ] PROUD
- [ ] HOPEFUL
- [ ] LOVING
- [ ] CONNECTED
- [ ] BALANCED
- [ ] JOYFUL
- [ ] RELAXED
- [ ] CREATIVE
- [ ] EXCITED
- [ ] _____

- [ ] NEUTRAL
- [ ] INSECURE
- [ ] DISCOURAGED
- [ ] DRAINED
- [ ] SAD
- [ ] SCARED
- [ ] ANGRY
- [ ] ANNOYED
- [ ] ANXIOUS
- [ ] STRESSED
- [ ] OVERWHELMED
- [ ] _____

A POSITIVE THOUGHT TO CARRY ME TO SLEEP:
_____
_____
_____

MORNING

DATE ___/___/___

TODAY'S FOCUS:
_____
_____
_____
_____

AN AFFIRMATION FOR TODAY:
_____
_____
_____
_____

WHAT I'M GRATEFUL FOR:
_____
_____
_____
_____
_____
_____
_____
_____
_____

WHAT I'M EXCITED ABOUT TODAY:
_____
_____
_____

HOW I'LL MAKE SPACE FOR GRATITUDE TODAY:
_____
_____
_____

EVENING

GOOD THINGS THAT HAPPENED TODAY:

THINGS I DID TO MAKE A POSITIVE DIFFERENCE TODAY:

HOW I FELT TODAY:

- [ ] HAPPY
- [ ] CONTENT
- [ ] PROUD
- [ ] HOPEFUL
- [ ] LOVING
- [ ] CONNECTED
- [ ] BALANCED
- [ ] JOYFUL
- [ ] RELAXED
- [ ] CREATIVE
- [ ] EXCITED
- [ ] _____

- [ ] NEUTRAL
- [ ] INSECURE
- [ ] DISCOURAGED
- [ ] DRAINED
- [ ] SAD
- [ ] SCARED
- [ ] ANGRY
- [ ] ANNOYED
- [ ] ANXIOUS
- [ ] STRESSED
- [ ] OVERWHELMED
- [ ] _____

A POSITIVE THOUGHT TO CARRY ME TO SLEEP:

MORNING

DATE ___/___/___

TODAY'S FOCUS:
_____
_____
_____
_____

AN AFFIRMATION FOR TODAY:
_____
_____
_____

WHAT I'M GRATEFUL FOR:
_____
_____
_____
_____
_____
_____
_____
_____
_____

WHAT I'M EXCITED ABOUT TODAY:
_____
_____
_____

HOW I'LL MAKE SPACE FOR GRATITUDE TODAY:
_____
_____
_____

EVENING

GOOD THINGS THAT HAPPENED TODAY:
_____
_____
_____
_____

THINGS I DID TO MAKE A POSITIVE DIFFERENCE TODAY:
_____
_____
_____
_____

HOW I FELT TODAY:

- ☐ HAPPY
- ☐ CONTENT
- ☐ PROUD
- ☐ HOPEFUL
- ☐ LOVING
- ☐ CONNECTED
- ☐ BALANCED
- ☐ JOYFUL
- ☐ RELAXED
- ☐ CREATIVE
- ☐ EXCITED
- ☐ _____

- ☐ NEUTRAL
- ☐ INSECURE
- ☐ DISCOURAGED
- ☐ DRAINED
- ☐ SAD
- ☐ SCARED
- ☐ ANGRY
- ☐ ANNOYED
- ☐ ANXIOUS
- ☐ STRESSED
- ☐ OVERWHELMED
- ☐ _____

A POSITIVE THOUGHT TO CARRY ME TO SLEEP:
_____
_____
_____

MORNING

DATE ___/___/___

TODAY'S FOCUS:
_____
_____
_____
_____

AN AFFIRMATION FOR TODAY:
_____
_____
_____
_____

WHAT I'M GRATEFUL FOR:
_____
_____
_____
_____
_____
_____
_____
_____
_____

WHAT I'M EXCITED ABOUT TODAY:
_____
_____
_____

HOW I'LL MAKE SPACE FOR GRATITUDE TODAY:
_____
_____
_____

EVENING

GOOD THINGS THAT HAPPENED TODAY:
_____
_____
_____
_____

THINGS I DID TO MAKE A POSITIVE DIFFERENCE TODAY:
_____
_____
_____
_____

HOW I FELT TODAY:

- ☐ HAPPY
- ☐ CONTENT
- ☐ PROUD
- ☐ HOPEFUL
- ☐ LOVING
- ☐ CONNECTED
- ☐ BALANCED
- ☐ JOYFUL
- ☐ RELAXED
- ☐ CREATIVE
- ☐ EXCITED
- ☐ _____

- ☐ NEUTRAL
- ☐ INSECURE
- ☐ DISCOURAGED
- ☐ DRAINED
- ☐ SAD
- ☐ SCARED
- ☐ ANGRY
- ☐ ANNOYED
- ☐ ANXIOUS
- ☐ STRESSED
- ☐ OVERWHELMED
- ☐ _____

_____
_____
_____
_____
_____
_____

A POSITIVE THOUGHT TO CARRY ME TO SLEEP:
_____
_____

MORNING

DATE ____/____/____

TODAY'S FOCUS:
_____
_____
_____
_____

AN AFFIRMATION FOR TODAY:
_____
_____
_____
_____

WHAT I'M GRATEFUL FOR:
_____
_____
_____
_____
_____
_____
_____
_____

WHAT I'M EXCITED ABOUT TODAY:
_____
_____
_____

HOW I'LL MAKE SPACE FOR GRATITUDE TODAY:
_____
_____
_____

EVENING

GOOD THINGS THAT HAPPENED TODAY:
___
___
___
___

THINGS I DID TO MAKE A POSITIVE DIFFERENCE TODAY:
___
___
___
___

HOW I FELT TODAY:

- ☐ HAPPY
- ☐ CONTENT
- ☐ PROUD
- ☐ HOPEFUL
- ☐ LOVING
- ☐ CONNECTED
- ☐ BALANCED
- ☐ JOYFUL
- ☐ RELAXED
- ☐ CREATIVE
- ☐ EXCITED
- ☐ _____

- ☐ NEUTRAL
- ☐ INSECURE
- ☐ DISCOURAGED
- ☐ DRAINED
- ☐ SAD
- ☐ SCARED
- ☐ ANGRY
- ☐ ANNOYED
- ☐ ANXIOUS
- ☐ STRESSED
- ☐ OVERWHELMED
- ☐ _____

A POSITIVE THOUGHT TO CARRY ME TO SLEEP:
___
___
___

MORNING

DATE ___/___/___

TODAY'S FOCUS:
_____
_____
_____
_____

AN AFFIRMATION FOR TODAY:
_____
_____
_____
_____

WHAT I'M GRATEFUL FOR:
_____
_____
_____
_____
_____
_____
_____
_____
_____
_____

WHAT I'M EXCITED ABOUT TODAY:
_____
_____
_____

HOW I'LL MAKE SPACE FOR GRATITUDE TODAY:
_____
_____

EVENING

GOOD THINGS THAT HAPPENED TODAY:

THINGS I DID TO MAKE A POSITIVE DIFFERENCE TODAY:

HOW I FELT TODAY:

- ☐ HAPPY
- ☐ CONTENT
- ☐ PROUD
- ☐ HOPEFUL
- ☐ LOVING
- ☐ CONNECTED
- ☐ BALANCED
- ☐ JOYFUL
- ☐ RELAXED
- ☐ CREATIVE
- ☐ EXCITED
- ☐ _____

- ☐ NEUTRAL
- ☐ INSECURE
- ☐ DISCOURAGED
- ☐ DRAINED
- ☐ SAD
- ☐ SCARED
- ☐ ANGRY
- ☐ ANNOYED
- ☐ ANXIOUS
- ☐ STRESSED
- ☐ OVERWHELMED
- ☐ _____

A POSITIVE THOUGHT TO CARRY ME TO SLEEP:

MORNING

DATE ___/___/___

TODAY'S FOCUS:

AN AFFIRMATION FOR TODAY:

WHAT I'M GRATEFUL FOR:

WHAT I'M EXCITED ABOUT TODAY:

HOW I'LL MAKE SPACE FOR GRATITUDE TODAY:

EVENING

GOOD THINGS THAT HAPPENED TODAY:
_____
_____
_____
_____

THINGS I DID TO MAKE A POSITIVE DIFFERENCE TODAY:
_____
_____
_____

HOW I FELT TODAY:

- ☐ HAPPY
- ☐ CONTENT
- ☐ PROUD
- ☐ HOPEFUL
- ☐ LOVING
- ☐ CONNECTED
- ☐ BALANCED
- ☐ JOYFUL
- ☐ RELAXED
- ☐ CREATIVE
- ☐ EXCITED
- ☐ _____

- ☐ NEUTRAL
- ☐ INSECURE
- ☐ DISCOURAGED
- ☐ DRAINED
- ☐ SAD
- ☐ SCARED
- ☐ ANGRY
- ☐ ANNOYED
- ☐ ANXIOUS
- ☐ STRESSED
- ☐ OVERWHELMED
- ☐ _____

A POSITIVE THOUGHT TO CARRY ME TO SLEEP:
_____
_____
_____

MORNING

DATE ___/___/___

TODAY'S FOCUS:
_____
_____
_____
_____

AN AFFIRMATION FOR TODAY:
_____
_____
_____

WHAT I'M GRATEFUL FOR:
_____
_____
_____
_____
_____
_____
_____
_____

WHAT I'M EXCITED ABOUT TODAY:
_____
_____
_____

HOW I'LL MAKE SPACE FOR GRATITUDE TODAY:
_____
_____
_____

EVENING

GOOD THINGS THAT HAPPENED TODAY:
___

THINGS I DID TO MAKE A POSITIVE DIFFERENCE TODAY:
___

HOW I FELT TODAY:

- ☐ HAPPY
- ☐ CONTENT
- ☐ PROUD
- ☐ HOPEFUL
- ☐ LOVING
- ☐ CONNECTED
- ☐ BALANCED
- ☐ JOYFUL
- ☐ RELAXED
- ☐ CREATIVE
- ☐ EXCITED
- ☐ _____

- ☐ NEUTRAL
- ☐ INSECURE
- ☐ DISCOURAGED
- ☐ DRAINED
- ☐ SAD
- ☐ SCARED
- ☐ ANGRY
- ☐ ANNOYED
- ☐ ANXIOUS
- ☐ STRESSED
- ☐ OVERWHELMED
- ☐ _____

A POSITIVE THOUGHT TO CARRY ME TO SLEEP:
___

MORNING

DATE ___/___/___

TODAY'S FOCUS:
_____
_____
_____
_____

AN AFFIRMATION FOR TODAY:
_____
_____
_____

WHAT I'M GRATEFUL FOR:
_____
_____
_____
_____
_____
_____
_____

WHAT I'M EXCITED ABOUT TODAY:
_____
_____
_____

HOW I'LL MAKE SPACE FOR GRATITUDE TODAY:
_____
_____
_____

EVENING

GOOD THINGS THAT HAPPENED TODAY:

_____
_____
_____
_____

THINGS I DID TO MAKE A POSITIVE DIFFERENCE TODAY:

_____
_____
_____
_____

HOW I FELT TODAY:

- ☐ HAPPY
- ☐ CONTENT
- ☐ PROUD
- ☐ HOPEFUL
- ☐ LOVING
- ☐ CONNECTED
- ☐ BALANCED
- ☐ JOYFUL
- ☐ RELAXED
- ☐ CREATIVE
- ☐ EXCITED
- ☐ _____

- ☐ NEUTRAL
- ☐ INSECURE
- ☐ DISCOURAGED
- ☐ DRAINED
- ☐ SAD
- ☐ SCARED
- ☐ ANGRY
- ☐ ANNOYED
- ☐ ANXIOUS
- ☐ STRESSED
- ☐ OVERWHELMED
- ☐ _____

A POSITIVE THOUGHT TO CARRY ME TO SLEEP:

_____
_____
_____

MORNING

DATE ____/____/____

TODAY'S FOCUS:
_____
_____
_____
_____

AN AFFIRMATION FOR TODAY:
_____
_____
_____
_____

WHAT I'M GRATEFUL FOR:
_____
_____
_____
_____
_____
_____
_____
_____
_____

WHAT I'M EXCITED ABOUT TODAY:
_____
_____
_____

HOW I'LL MAKE SPACE FOR GRATITUDE TODAY:
_____
_____
_____

EVENING

GOOD THINGS THAT HAPPENED TODAY:
_____
_____
_____

THINGS I DID TO MAKE A POSITIVE DIFFERENCE TODAY:
_____
_____
_____

HOW I FELT TODAY:

- ☐ HAPPY
- ☐ CONTENT
- ☐ PROUD
- ☐ HOPEFUL
- ☐ LOVING
- ☐ CONNECTED
- ☐ BALANCED
- ☐ JOYFUL
- ☐ RELAXED
- ☐ CREATIVE
- ☐ EXCITED
- ☐ _____

- ☐ NEUTRAL
- ☐ INSECURE
- ☐ DISCOURAGED
- ☐ DRAINED
- ☐ SAD
- ☐ SCARED
- ☐ ANGRY
- ☐ ANNOYED
- ☐ ANXIOUS
- ☐ STRESSED
- ☐ OVERWHELMED
- ☐ _____

_____
_____
_____
_____
_____
_____

A POSITIVE THOUGHT TO CARRY ME TO SLEEP:
_____
_____
_____

MORNING

DATE ___/___/___

TODAY'S FOCUS:
_____
_____
_____
_____

AN AFFIRMATION FOR TODAY:
_____
_____
_____

WHAT I'M GRATEFUL FOR:
_____
_____
_____
_____
_____
_____
_____
_____

WHAT I'M EXCITED ABOUT TODAY:
_____
_____

HOW I'LL MAKE SPACE FOR GRATITUDE TODAY:
_____
_____

EVENING

GOOD THINGS THAT HAPPENED TODAY:
_____
_____
_____
_____

THINGS I DID TO MAKE A POSITIVE DIFFERENCE TODAY:
_____
_____
_____
_____

HOW I FELT TODAY:

- ☐ HAPPY
- ☐ CONTENT
- ☐ PROUD
- ☐ HOPEFUL
- ☐ LOVING
- ☐ CONNECTED
- ☐ BALANCED
- ☐ JOYFUL
- ☐ RELAXED
- ☐ CREATIVE
- ☐ EXCITED
- ☐ _____

- ☐ NEUTRAL
- ☐ INSECURE
- ☐ DISCOURAGED
- ☐ DRAINED
- ☐ SAD
- ☐ SCARED
- ☐ ANGRY
- ☐ ANNOYED
- ☐ ANXIOUS
- ☐ STRESSED
- ☐ OVERWHELMED
- ☐ _____

A POSITIVE THOUGHT TO CARRY ME TO SLEEP:
_____
_____
_____

MORNING

DATE ___/___/___

TODAY'S FOCUS:
_____
_____
_____
_____

AN AFFIRMATION FOR TODAY:
_____
_____
_____
_____

WHAT I'M GRATEFUL FOR:
_____
_____
_____
_____
_____
_____
_____
_____

WHAT I'M EXCITED ABOUT TODAY:
_____
_____

HOW I'LL MAKE SPACE FOR GRATITUDE TODAY:
_____
_____

EVENING

GOOD THINGS THAT HAPPENED TODAY:
_____
_____
_____
_____

THINGS I DID TO MAKE A POSITIVE DIFFERENCE TODAY:
_____
_____
_____
_____

HOW I FELT TODAY:

- ☐ HAPPY
- ☐ CONTENT
- ☐ PROUD
- ☐ HOPEFUL
- ☐ LOVING
- ☐ CONNECTED
- ☐ BALANCED
- ☐ JOYFUL
- ☐ RELAXED
- ☐ CREATIVE
- ☐ EXCITED
- ☐ _____

- ☐ NEUTRAL
- ☐ INSECURE
- ☐ DISCOURAGED
- ☐ DRAINED
- ☐ SAD
- ☐ SCARED
- ☐ ANGRY
- ☐ ANNOYED
- ☐ ANXIOUS
- ☐ STRESSED
- ☐ OVERWHELMED
- ☐ _____

A POSITIVE THOUGHT TO CARRY ME TO SLEEP:
_____
_____
_____

MORNING

DATE ____/____/____

TODAY'S FOCUS:
_____
_____
_____
_____

AN AFFIRMATION FOR TODAY:
_____
_____
_____
_____

WHAT I'M GRATEFUL FOR:
_____
_____
_____
_____
_____
_____
_____
_____

WHAT I'M EXCITED ABOUT TODAY:
_____
_____
_____

HOW I'LL MAKE SPACE FOR GRATITUDE TODAY:
_____
_____
_____

EVENING

GOOD THINGS THAT HAPPENED TODAY:

_____
_____
_____

THINGS I DID TO MAKE A POSITIVE DIFFERENCE TODAY:

_____
_____
_____

HOW I FELT TODAY:

- ☐ HAPPY
- ☐ CONTENT
- ☐ PROUD
- ☐ HOPEFUL
- ☐ LOVING
- ☐ CONNECTED
- ☐ BALANCED
- ☐ JOYFUL
- ☐ RELAXED
- ☐ CREATIVE
- ☐ EXCITED
- ☐ _____

- ☐ NEUTRAL
- ☐ INSECURE
- ☐ DISCOURAGED
- ☐ DRAINED
- ☐ SAD
- ☐ SCARED
- ☐ ANGRY
- ☐ ANNOYED
- ☐ ANXIOUS
- ☐ STRESSED
- ☐ OVERWHELMED
- ☐ _____

A POSITIVE THOUGHT TO CARRY ME TO SLEEP:

_____
_____

MORNING

DATE ___/___/___

TODAY'S FOCUS:
_____
_____
_____
_____

AN AFFIRMATION FOR TODAY:
_____
_____
_____

WHAT I'M GRATEFUL FOR:
_____
_____
_____
_____
_____
_____
_____
_____
_____

WHAT I'M EXCITED ABOUT TODAY:
_____
_____
_____

HOW I'LL MAKE SPACE FOR GRATITUDE TODAY:
_____
_____
_____

EVENING

GOOD THINGS THAT HAPPENED TODAY:
_____
_____
_____
_____

THINGS I DID TO MAKE A POSITIVE DIFFERENCE TODAY:
_____
_____
_____
_____

HOW I FELT TODAY:

- ☐ HAPPY
- ☐ CONTENT
- ☐ PROUD
- ☐ HOPEFUL
- ☐ LOVING
- ☐ CONNECTED
- ☐ BALANCED
- ☐ JOYFUL
- ☐ RELAXED
- ☐ CREATIVE
- ☐ EXCITED
- ☐ _____

- ☐ NEUTRAL
- ☐ INSECURE
- ☐ DISCOURAGED
- ☐ DRAINED
- ☐ SAD
- ☐ SCARED
- ☐ ANGRY
- ☐ ANNOYED
- ☐ ANXIOUS
- ☐ STRESSED
- ☐ OVERWHELMED
- ☐ _____

_____
_____
_____
_____
_____
_____

A POSITIVE THOUGHT TO CARRY ME TO SLEEP:
_____
_____
_____

MORNING

DATE ___/___/___

TODAY'S FOCUS:
_____
_____
_____
_____

AN AFFIRMATION FOR TODAY:
_____
_____
_____
_____

WHAT I'M GRATEFUL FOR:
_____
_____
_____
_____
_____
_____
_____
_____
_____

WHAT I'M EXCITED ABOUT TODAY:
_____
_____

HOW I'LL MAKE SPACE FOR GRATITUDE TODAY:
_____
_____
_____

EVENING

GOOD THINGS THAT HAPPENED TODAY:
_____
_____
_____
_____

THINGS I DID TO MAKE A POSITIVE DIFFERENCE TODAY:
_____
_____
_____
_____

HOW I FELT TODAY:

- ☐ HAPPY
- ☐ CONTENT
- ☐ PROUD
- ☐ HOPEFUL
- ☐ LOVING
- ☐ CONNECTED
- ☐ BALANCED
- ☐ JOYFUL
- ☐ RELAXED
- ☐ CREATIVE
- ☐ EXCITED
- ☐ _____

- ☐ NEUTRAL
- ☐ INSECURE
- ☐ DISCOURAGED
- ☐ DRAINED
- ☐ SAD
- ☐ SCARED
- ☐ ANGRY
- ☐ ANNOYED
- ☐ ANXIOUS
- ☐ STRESSED
- ☐ OVERWHELMED
- ☐ _____

A POSITIVE THOUGHT TO CARRY ME TO SLEEP:
_____
_____
_____

MORNING

DATE ___/___/___

TODAY'S FOCUS:
_____
_____
_____
_____

AN AFFIRMATION FOR TODAY:
_____
_____
_____
_____

WHAT I'M GRATEFUL FOR:
_____
_____
_____
_____
_____
_____
_____
_____
_____

WHAT I'M EXCITED ABOUT TODAY:
_____
_____
_____

HOW I'LL MAKE SPACE FOR GRATITUDE TODAY:
_____
_____
_____

EVENING

GOOD THINGS THAT HAPPENED TODAY:
_____
_____
_____
_____

THINGS I DID TO MAKE A POSITIVE DIFFERENCE TODAY:
_____
_____
_____
_____

HOW I FELT TODAY:

- ☐ HAPPY
- ☐ CONTENT
- ☐ PROUD
- ☐ HOPEFUL
- ☐ LOVING
- ☐ CONNECTED
- ☐ BALANCED
- ☐ JOYFUL
- ☐ RELAXED
- ☐ CREATIVE
- ☐ EXCITED
- ☐ _____

- ☐ NEUTRAL
- ☐ INSECURE
- ☐ DISCOURAGED
- ☐ DRAINED
- ☐ SAD
- ☐ SCARED
- ☐ ANGRY
- ☐ ANNOYED
- ☐ ANXIOUS
- ☐ STRESSED
- ☐ OVERWHELMED
- ☐ _____

A POSITIVE THOUGHT TO CARRY ME TO SLEEP:
_____
_____
_____

MORNING

DATE ___/___/___

TODAY'S FOCUS:

AN AFFIRMATION FOR TODAY:

WHAT I'M GRATEFUL FOR:

WHAT I'M EXCITED ABOUT TODAY:

HOW I'LL MAKE SPACE FOR GRATITUDE TODAY:

EVENING

GOOD THINGS THAT HAPPENED TODAY:

_____
_____
_____
_____

THINGS I DID TO MAKE A POSITIVE DIFFERENCE TODAY:

_____
_____
_____
_____

HOW I FELT TODAY:

- ☐ HAPPY
- ☐ CONTENT
- ☐ PROUD
- ☐ HOPEFUL
- ☐ LOVING
- ☐ CONNECTED
- ☐ BALANCED
- ☐ JOYFUL
- ☐ RELAXED
- ☐ CREATIVE
- ☐ EXCITED
- ☐ _____

- ☐ NEUTRAL
- ☐ INSECURE
- ☐ DISCOURAGED
- ☐ DRAINED
- ☐ SAD
- ☐ SCARED
- ☐ ANGRY
- ☐ ANNOYED
- ☐ ANXIOUS
- ☐ STRESSED
- ☐ OVERWHELMED
- ☐ _____

_____
_____
_____
_____
_____
_____

A POSITIVE THOUGHT TO CARRY ME TO SLEEP:

_____
_____
_____

MORNING

DATE ___/___/___

TODAY'S FOCUS:
_____
_____
_____

AN AFFIRMATION FOR TODAY:
_____
_____
_____

WHAT I'M GRATEFUL FOR:
_____
_____
_____
_____
_____
_____
_____

WHAT I'M EXCITED ABOUT TODAY:
_____
_____
_____

HOW I'LL MAKE SPACE FOR GRATITUDE TODAY:
_____
_____
_____

EVENING

GOOD THINGS THAT HAPPENED TODAY:
_____
_____
_____
_____

THINGS I DID TO MAKE A POSITIVE DIFFERENCE TODAY:
_____
_____
_____
_____

HOW I FELT TODAY:

- ☐ HAPPY
- ☐ CONTENT
- ☐ PROUD
- ☐ HOPEFUL
- ☐ LOVING
- ☐ CONNECTED
- ☐ BALANCED
- ☐ JOYFUL
- ☐ RELAXED
- ☐ CREATIVE
- ☐ EXCITED
- ☐ _____

- ☐ NEUTRAL
- ☐ INSECURE
- ☐ DISCOURAGED
- ☐ DRAINED
- ☐ SAD
- ☐ SCARED
- ☐ ANGRY
- ☐ ANNOYED
- ☐ ANXIOUS
- ☐ STRESSED
- ☐ OVERWHELMED
- ☐ _____

A POSITIVE THOUGHT TO CARRY ME TO SLEEP:
_____
_____
_____

MORNING

DATE ____/____/____

TODAY'S FOCUS:
_____
_____
_____
_____

AN AFFIRMATION FOR TODAY:
_____
_____
_____
_____

WHAT I'M GRATEFUL FOR:
_____
_____
_____
_____
_____
_____
_____
_____
_____

WHAT I'M EXCITED ABOUT TODAY:
_____
_____
_____

HOW I'LL MAKE SPACE FOR GRATITUDE TODAY:
_____
_____
_____

EVENING

GOOD THINGS THAT HAPPENED TODAY:

THINGS I DID TO MAKE A POSITIVE DIFFERENCE TODAY:

HOW I FELT TODAY:

- ☐ HAPPY
- ☐ CONTENT
- ☐ PROUD
- ☐ HOPEFUL
- ☐ LOVING
- ☐ CONNECTED
- ☐ BALANCED
- ☐ JOYFUL
- ☐ RELAXED
- ☐ CREATIVE
- ☐ EXCITED
- ☐ _____

- ☐ NEUTRAL
- ☐ INSECURE
- ☐ DISCOURAGED
- ☐ DRAINED
- ☐ SAD
- ☐ SCARED
- ☐ ANGRY
- ☐ ANNOYED
- ☐ ANXIOUS
- ☐ STRESSED
- ☐ OVERWHELMED
- ☐ _____

A POSITIVE THOUGHT TO CARRY ME TO SLEEP:

MORNING

DATE ____/____/____

TODAY'S FOCUS:
_____
_____
_____
_____

AN AFFIRMATION FOR TODAY:
_____
_____
_____
_____

WHAT I'M GRATEFUL FOR:
_____
_____
_____
_____
_____
_____
_____
_____
_____

WHAT I'M EXCITED ABOUT TODAY:
_____
_____
_____

HOW I'LL MAKE SPACE FOR GRATITUDE TODAY:
_____
_____
_____

EVENING

GOOD THINGS THAT HAPPENED TODAY:
_____
_____
_____
_____

THINGS I DID TO MAKE A POSITIVE DIFFERENCE TODAY:
_____
_____
_____
_____

HOW I FELT TODAY:

- ☐ HAPPY
- ☐ CONTENT
- ☐ PROUD
- ☐ HOPEFUL
- ☐ LOVING
- ☐ CONNECTED
- ☐ BALANCED
- ☐ JOYFUL
- ☐ RELAXED
- ☐ CREATIVE
- ☐ EXCITED
- ☐ _____

- ☐ NEUTRAL
- ☐ INSECURE
- ☐ DISCOURAGED
- ☐ DRAINED
- ☐ SAD
- ☐ SCARED
- ☐ ANGRY
- ☐ ANNOYED
- ☐ ANXIOUS
- ☐ STRESSED
- ☐ OVERWHELMED
- ☐ _____

A POSITIVE THOUGHT TO CARRY ME TO SLEEP:
_____
_____
_____

MORNING

DATE ___/___/___

TODAY'S FOCUS:
_____
_____
_____
_____

AN AFFIRMATION FOR TODAY:
_____
_____
_____
_____

WHAT I'M GRATEFUL FOR:
_____
_____
_____
_____
_____
_____
_____
_____

WHAT I'M EXCITED ABOUT TODAY:
_____
_____
_____

HOW I'LL MAKE SPACE FOR GRATITUDE TODAY:
_____
_____
_____

EVENING

GOOD THINGS THAT HAPPENED TODAY:

THINGS I DID TO MAKE A POSITIVE DIFFERENCE TODAY:

HOW I FELT TODAY:

- ☐ HAPPY
- ☐ CONTENT
- ☐ PROUD
- ☐ HOPEFUL
- ☐ LOVING
- ☐ CONNECTED
- ☐ BALANCED
- ☐ JOYFUL
- ☐ RELAXED
- ☐ CREATIVE
- ☐ EXCITED
- ☐ _____

- ☐ NEUTRAL
- ☐ INSECURE
- ☐ DISCOURAGED
- ☐ DRAINED
- ☐ SAD
- ☐ SCARED
- ☐ ANGRY
- ☐ ANNOYED
- ☐ ANXIOUS
- ☐ STRESSED
- ☐ OVERWHELMED
- ☐ _____

A POSITIVE THOUGHT TO CARRY ME TO SLEEP:

MORNING

DATE ___/___/___

TODAY'S FOCUS:
_____
_____
_____
_____

AN AFFIRMATION FOR TODAY:
_____
_____
_____
_____

WHAT I'M GRATEFUL FOR:
_____
_____
_____
_____
_____
_____
_____
_____

WHAT I'M EXCITED ABOUT TODAY:
_____
_____
_____

HOW I'LL MAKE SPACE FOR GRATITUDE TODAY:
_____
_____
_____

EVENING

GOOD THINGS THAT HAPPENED TODAY:
___
___
___
___

THINGS I DID TO MAKE A POSITIVE DIFFERENCE TODAY:
___
___
___
___

HOW I FELT TODAY:

- ☐ HAPPY
- ☐ CONTENT
- ☐ PROUD
- ☐ HOPEFUL
- ☐ LOVING
- ☐ CONNECTED
- ☐ BALANCED
- ☐ JOYFUL
- ☐ RELAXED
- ☐ CREATIVE
- ☐ EXCITED
- ☐ _____

- ☐ NEUTRAL
- ☐ INSECURE
- ☐ DISCOURAGED
- ☐ DRAINED
- ☐ SAD
- ☐ SCARED
- ☐ ANGRY
- ☐ ANNOYED
- ☐ ANXIOUS
- ☐ STRESSED
- ☐ OVERWHELMED
- ☐ _____

A POSITIVE THOUGHT TO CARRY ME TO SLEEP:
___
___
___

MORNING

DATE ___/___/___

TODAY'S FOCUS:
_____
_____
_____
_____

AN AFFIRMATION FOR TODAY:
_____
_____
_____

WHAT I'M GRATEFUL FOR:
_____
_____
_____
_____
_____
_____
_____
_____
_____

WHAT I'M EXCITED ABOUT TODAY:
_____
_____
_____

HOW I'LL MAKE SPACE FOR GRATITUDE TODAY:
_____
_____
_____

EVENING

GOOD THINGS THAT HAPPENED TODAY:
_____
_____
_____
_____

THINGS I DID TO MAKE A POSITIVE DIFFERENCE TODAY:
_____
_____
_____
_____

HOW I FELT TODAY:

- ☐ HAPPY
- ☐ CONTENT
- ☐ PROUD
- ☐ HOPEFUL
- ☐ LOVING
- ☐ CONNECTED
- ☐ BALANCED
- ☐ JOYFUL
- ☐ RELAXED
- ☐ CREATIVE
- ☐ EXCITED
- ☐ _____

- ☐ NEUTRAL
- ☐ INSECURE
- ☐ DISCOURAGED
- ☐ DRAINED
- ☐ SAD
- ☐ SCARED
- ☐ ANGRY
- ☐ ANNOYED
- ☐ ANXIOUS
- ☐ STRESSED
- ☐ OVERWHELMED
- ☐ _____

A POSITIVE THOUGHT TO CARRY ME TO SLEEP:
_____
_____
_____

MORNING

DATE ___/___/___

TODAY'S FOCUS:
_____
_____
_____
_____

AN AFFIRMATION FOR TODAY:
_____
_____
_____

WHAT I'M GRATEFUL FOR:
_____
_____
_____
_____
_____
_____
_____
_____

WHAT I'M EXCITED ABOUT TODAY:
_____
_____
_____

HOW I'LL MAKE SPACE FOR GRATITUDE TODAY:
_____
_____
_____

EVENING

GOOD THINGS THAT HAPPENED TODAY:
_____
_____
_____

THINGS I DID TO MAKE A POSITIVE DIFFERENCE TODAY:
_____
_____
_____

HOW I FELT TODAY:

- ☐ HAPPY
- ☐ CONTENT
- ☐ PROUD
- ☐ HOPEFUL
- ☐ LOVING
- ☐ CONNECTED
- ☐ BALANCED
- ☐ JOYFUL
- ☐ RELAXED
- ☐ CREATIVE
- ☐ EXCITED
- ☐ _____

- ☐ NEUTRAL
- ☐ INSECURE
- ☐ DISCOURAGED
- ☐ DRAINED
- ☐ SAD
- ☐ SCARED
- ☐ ANGRY
- ☐ ANNOYED
- ☐ ANXIOUS
- ☐ STRESSED
- ☐ OVERWHELMED
- ☐ _____

A POSITIVE THOUGHT TO CARRY ME TO SLEEP:
_____
_____
_____

MORNING

DATE ___/___/___

TODAY'S FOCUS:

AN AFFIRMATION FOR TODAY:

WHAT I'M GRATEFUL FOR:

WHAT I'M EXCITED ABOUT TODAY:

HOW I'LL MAKE SPACE FOR GRATITUDE TODAY:

EVENING

GOOD THINGS THAT HAPPENED TODAY:
_____
_____
_____
_____

THINGS I DID TO MAKE A POSITIVE DIFFERENCE TODAY:
_____
_____
_____
_____

HOW I FELT TODAY:

- [ ] HAPPY
- [ ] CONTENT
- [ ] PROUD
- [ ] HOPEFUL
- [ ] LOVING
- [ ] CONNECTED
- [ ] BALANCED
- [ ] JOYFUL
- [ ] RELAXED
- [ ] CREATIVE
- [ ] EXCITED
- [ ] _____

- [ ] NEUTRAL
- [ ] INSECURE
- [ ] DISCOURAGED
- [ ] DRAINED
- [ ] SAD
- [ ] SCARED
- [ ] ANGRY
- [ ] ANNOYED
- [ ] ANXIOUS
- [ ] STRESSED
- [ ] OVERWHELMED
- [ ] _____

A POSITIVE THOUGHT TO CARRY ME TO SLEEP:
_____
_____
_____

MORNING

DATE ___/___/___

TODAY'S FOCUS:
_____
_____
_____
_____

AN AFFIRMATION FOR TODAY:
_____
_____
_____
_____

WHAT I'M GRATEFUL FOR:
_____
_____
_____
_____
_____
_____
_____
_____
_____

WHAT I'M EXCITED ABOUT TODAY:
_____
_____
_____

HOW I'LL MAKE SPACE FOR GRATITUDE TODAY:
_____
_____
_____

EVENING

GOOD THINGS THAT HAPPENED TODAY:

THINGS I DID TO MAKE A POSITIVE DIFFERENCE TODAY:

HOW I FELT TODAY:

- ☐ HAPPY
- ☐ CONTENT
- ☐ PROUD
- ☐ HOPEFUL
- ☐ LOVING
- ☐ CONNECTED
- ☐ BALANCED
- ☐ JOYFUL
- ☐ RELAXED
- ☐ CREATIVE
- ☐ EXCITED
- ☐ _____

- ☐ NEUTRAL
- ☐ INSECURE
- ☐ DISCOURAGED
- ☐ DRAINED
- ☐ SAD
- ☐ SCARED
- ☐ ANGRY
- ☐ ANNOYED
- ☐ ANXIOUS
- ☐ STRESSED
- ☐ OVERWHELMED
- ☐ _____

A POSITIVE THOUGHT TO CARRY ME TO SLEEP:

MORNING

DATE ___/___/___

TODAY'S FOCUS:
_____
_____
_____
_____

AN AFFIRMATION FOR TODAY:
_____
_____
_____

WHAT I'M GRATEFUL FOR:
_____
_____
_____
_____
_____
_____
_____
_____

WHAT I'M EXCITED ABOUT TODAY:
_____
_____
_____

HOW I'LL MAKE SPACE FOR GRATITUDE TODAY:
_____
_____
_____

EVENING

GOOD THINGS THAT HAPPENED TODAY:

THINGS I DID TO MAKE A POSITIVE DIFFERENCE TODAY:

HOW I FELT TODAY:

- ☐ HAPPY
- ☐ CONTENT
- ☐ PROUD
- ☐ HOPEFUL
- ☐ LOVING
- ☐ CONNECTED
- ☐ BALANCED
- ☐ JOYFUL
- ☐ RELAXED
- ☐ CREATIVE
- ☐ EXCITED
- ☐ _____

- ☐ NEUTRAL
- ☐ INSECURE
- ☐ DISCOURAGED
- ☐ DRAINED
- ☐ SAD
- ☐ SCARED
- ☐ ANGRY
- ☐ ANNOYED
- ☐ ANXIOUS
- ☐ STRESSED
- ☐ OVERWHELMED
- ☐ _____

A POSITIVE THOUGHT TO CARRY ME TO SLEEP:

MORNING

DATE ___/___/___

TODAY'S FOCUS:

AN AFFIRMATION FOR TODAY:

WHAT I'M GRATEFUL FOR:

WHAT I'M EXCITED ABOUT TODAY:

HOW I'LL MAKE SPACE FOR GRATITUDE TODAY:

EVENING

GOOD THINGS THAT HAPPENED TODAY:
_____
_____
_____
_____

THINGS I DID TO MAKE A POSITIVE DIFFERENCE TODAY:
_____
_____
_____
_____

HOW I FELT TODAY:

- ☐ HAPPY
- ☐ CONTENT
- ☐ PROUD
- ☐ HOPEFUL
- ☐ LOVING
- ☐ CONNECTED
- ☐ BALANCED
- ☐ JOYFUL
- ☐ RELAXED
- ☐ CREATIVE
- ☐ EXCITED
- ☐ _____

- ☐ NEUTRAL
- ☐ INSECURE
- ☐ DISCOURAGED
- ☐ DRAINED
- ☐ SAD
- ☐ SCARED
- ☐ ANGRY
- ☐ ANNOYED
- ☐ ANXIOUS
- ☐ STRESSED
- ☐ OVERWHELMED
- ☐ _____

A POSITIVE THOUGHT TO CARRY ME TO SLEEP:
_____
_____
_____

MORNING

DATE ___/___/___

TODAY'S FOCUS:
_____
_____
_____

AN AFFIRMATION FOR TODAY:
_____
_____
_____

WHAT I'M GRATEFUL FOR:
_____
_____
_____
_____
_____
_____
_____
_____

WHAT I'M EXCITED ABOUT TODAY:
_____
_____
_____

HOW I'LL MAKE SPACE FOR GRATITUDE TODAY:
_____
_____
_____

EVENING

GOOD THINGS THAT HAPPENED TODAY:

THINGS I DID TO MAKE A POSITIVE DIFFERENCE TODAY:

HOW I FELT TODAY:

- ☐ HAPPY
- ☐ CONTENT
- ☐ PROUD
- ☐ HOPEFUL
- ☐ LOVING
- ☐ CONNECTED
- ☐ BALANCED
- ☐ JOYFUL
- ☐ RELAXED
- ☐ CREATIVE
- ☐ EXCITED
- ☐ _____

- ☐ NEUTRAL
- ☐ INSECURE
- ☐ DISCOURAGED
- ☐ DRAINED
- ☐ SAD
- ☐ SCARED
- ☐ ANGRY
- ☐ ANNOYED
- ☐ ANXIOUS
- ☐ STRESSED
- ☐ OVERWHELMED
- ☐ _____

A POSITIVE THOUGHT TO CARRY ME TO SLEEP:

MORNING

DATE ___/___/___

TODAY'S FOCUS:
_____
_____
_____
_____

AN AFFIRMATION FOR TODAY:
_____
_____
_____
_____

WHAT I'M GRATEFUL FOR:
_____
_____
_____
_____
_____
_____
_____
_____

WHAT I'M EXCITED ABOUT TODAY:
_____
_____
_____

HOW I'LL MAKE SPACE FOR GRATITUDE TODAY:
_____
_____
_____

EVENING

GOOD THINGS THAT HAPPENED TODAY:

THINGS I DID TO MAKE A POSITIVE DIFFERENCE TODAY:

HOW I FELT TODAY:

- ☐ HAPPY
- ☐ CONTENT
- ☐ PROUD
- ☐ HOPEFUL
- ☐ LOVING
- ☐ CONNECTED
- ☐ BALANCED
- ☐ JOYFUL
- ☐ RELAXED
- ☐ CREATIVE
- ☐ EXCITED
- ☐ _____

- ☐ NEUTRAL
- ☐ INSECURE
- ☐ DISCOURAGED
- ☐ DRAINED
- ☐ SAD
- ☐ SCARED
- ☐ ANGRY
- ☐ ANNOYED
- ☐ ANXIOUS
- ☐ STRESSED
- ☐ OVERWHELMED
- ☐ _____

A POSITIVE THOUGHT TO CARRY ME TO SLEEP:

MORNING

DATE ___/___/___

TODAY'S FOCUS:

AN AFFIRMATION FOR TODAY:

WHAT I'M GRATEFUL FOR:

WHAT I'M EXCITED ABOUT TODAY:

HOW I'LL MAKE SPACE FOR GRATITUDE TODAY:

EVENING

GOOD THINGS THAT HAPPENED TODAY:
_____
_____
_____
_____

THINGS I DID TO MAKE A POSITIVE DIFFERENCE TODAY:
_____
_____
_____
_____

HOW I FELT TODAY:

- ☐ HAPPY
- ☐ CONTENT
- ☐ PROUD
- ☐ HOPEFUL
- ☐ LOVING
- ☐ CONNECTED
- ☐ BALANCED
- ☐ JOYFUL
- ☐ RELAXED
- ☐ CREATIVE
- ☐ EXCITED
- ☐ _____

- ☐ NEUTRAL
- ☐ INSECURE
- ☐ DISCOURAGED
- ☐ DRAINED
- ☐ SAD
- ☐ SCARED
- ☐ ANGRY
- ☐ ANNOYED
- ☐ ANXIOUS
- ☐ STRESSED
- ☐ OVERWHELMED
- ☐ _____

A POSITIVE THOUGHT TO CARRY ME TO SLEEP:
_____
_____
_____

MORNING

DATE ___/___/___

TODAY'S FOCUS:
_____
_____
_____
_____

AN AFFIRMATION FOR TODAY:
_____
_____
_____

WHAT I'M GRATEFUL FOR:
_____
_____
_____
_____
_____
_____
_____
_____
_____

WHAT I'M EXCITED ABOUT TODAY:
_____
_____
_____

HOW I'LL MAKE SPACE FOR GRATITUDE TODAY:
_____
_____
_____

EVENING

GOOD THINGS THAT HAPPENED TODAY:
_____
_____
_____
_____

THINGS I DID TO MAKE A POSITIVE DIFFERENCE TODAY:
_____
_____
_____
_____

HOW I FELT TODAY:

- ☐ HAPPY
- ☐ CONTENT
- ☐ PROUD
- ☐ HOPEFUL
- ☐ LOVING
- ☐ CONNECTED
- ☐ BALANCED
- ☐ JOYFUL
- ☐ RELAXED
- ☐ CREATIVE
- ☐ EXCITED
- ☐ _____

- ☐ NEUTRAL
- ☐ INSECURE
- ☐ DISCOURAGED
- ☐ DRAINED
- ☐ SAD
- ☐ SCARED
- ☐ ANGRY
- ☐ ANNOYED
- ☐ ANXIOUS
- ☐ STRESSED
- ☐ OVERWHELMED
- ☐ _____

A POSITIVE THOUGHT TO CARRY ME TO SLEEP:
_____
_____
_____

MORNING

DATE ___/___/___

TODAY'S FOCUS:

AN AFFIRMATION FOR TODAY:

WHAT I'M GRATEFUL FOR:

WHAT I'M EXCITED ABOUT TODAY:

HOW I'LL MAKE SPACE FOR GRATITUDE TODAY:

EVENING

GOOD THINGS THAT HAPPENED TODAY:
_____
_____
_____
_____

THINGS I DID TO MAKE A POSITIVE DIFFERENCE TODAY:
_____
_____
_____
_____

HOW I FELT TODAY:

- ☐ HAPPY
- ☐ CONTENT
- ☐ PROUD
- ☐ HOPEFUL
- ☐ LOVING
- ☐ CONNECTED
- ☐ BALANCED
- ☐ JOYFUL
- ☐ RELAXED
- ☐ CREATIVE
- ☐ EXCITED
- ☐ _____

- ☐ NEUTRAL
- ☐ INSECURE
- ☐ DISCOURAGED
- ☐ DRAINED
- ☐ SAD
- ☐ SCARED
- ☐ ANGRY
- ☐ ANNOYED
- ☐ ANXIOUS
- ☐ STRESSED
- ☐ OVERWHELMED
- ☐ _____

A POSITIVE THOUGHT TO CARRY ME TO SLEEP:
_____
_____
_____

MORNING

DATE ___/___/___

TODAY'S FOCUS:
_____
_____
_____
_____

AN AFFIRMATION FOR TODAY:
_____
_____
_____
_____

WHAT I'M GRATEFUL FOR:
_____
_____
_____
_____
_____
_____
_____
_____
_____

WHAT I'M EXCITED ABOUT TODAY:
_____
_____
_____

HOW I'LL MAKE SPACE FOR GRATITUDE TODAY:
_____
_____
_____

EVENING

GOOD THINGS THAT HAPPENED TODAY:

THINGS I DID TO MAKE A POSITIVE DIFFERENCE TODAY:

HOW I FELT TODAY:

- [ ] HAPPY
- [ ] CONTENT
- [ ] PROUD
- [ ] HOPEFUL
- [ ] LOVING
- [ ] CONNECTED
- [ ] BALANCED
- [ ] JOYFUL
- [ ] RELAXED
- [ ] CREATIVE
- [ ] EXCITED
- [ ] _____

- [ ] NEUTRAL
- [ ] INSECURE
- [ ] DISCOURAGED
- [ ] DRAINED
- [ ] SAD
- [ ] SCARED
- [ ] ANGRY
- [ ] ANNOYED
- [ ] ANXIOUS
- [ ] STRESSED
- [ ] OVERWHELMED
- [ ] _____

A POSITIVE THOUGHT TO CARRY ME TO SLEEP:

MORNING

DATE ____/____/____

TODAY'S FOCUS:
_____
_____
_____
_____

AN AFFIRMATION FOR TODAY:
_____
_____
_____

WHAT I'M GRATEFUL FOR:
_____
_____
_____
_____
_____
_____
_____
_____
_____

WHAT I'M EXCITED ABOUT TODAY:
_____
_____
_____

HOW I'LL MAKE SPACE FOR GRATITUDE TODAY:
_____
_____
_____

EVENING

GOOD THINGS THAT HAPPENED TODAY:
_____
_____
_____
_____

THINGS I DID TO MAKE A POSITIVE DIFFERENCE TODAY:
_____
_____
_____
_____

HOW I FELT TODAY:

- ☐ HAPPY
- ☐ CONTENT
- ☐ PROUD
- ☐ HOPEFUL
- ☐ LOVING
- ☐ CONNECTED
- ☐ BALANCED
- ☐ JOYFUL
- ☐ RELAXED
- ☐ CREATIVE
- ☐ EXCITED
- ☐ _____

- ☐ NEUTRAL
- ☐ INSECURE
- ☐ DISCOURAGED
- ☐ DRAINED
- ☐ SAD
- ☐ SCARED
- ☐ ANGRY
- ☐ ANNOYED
- ☐ ANXIOUS
- ☐ STRESSED
- ☐ OVERWHELMED
- ☐ _____

A POSITIVE THOUGHT TO CARRY ME TO SLEEP:
_____
_____
_____

MORNING

DATE ___/___/___

TODAY'S FOCUS:
_____
_____
_____
_____

AN AFFIRMATION FOR TODAY:
_____
_____
_____
_____

WHAT I'M GRATEFUL FOR:
_____
_____
_____
_____
_____
_____
_____
_____
_____

WHAT I'M EXCITED ABOUT TODAY:
_____
_____
_____

HOW I'LL MAKE SPACE FOR GRATITUDE TODAY:
_____
_____
_____

EVENING

GOOD THINGS THAT HAPPENED TODAY:
_____
_____
_____
_____

THINGS I DID TO MAKE A POSITIVE DIFFERENCE TODAY:
_____
_____
_____
_____

HOW I FELT TODAY:

- ☐ HAPPY
- ☐ CONTENT
- ☐ PROUD
- ☐ HOPEFUL
- ☐ LOVING
- ☐ CONNECTED
- ☐ BALANCED
- ☐ JOYFUL
- ☐ RELAXED
- ☐ CREATIVE
- ☐ EXCITED
- ☐ _____

- ☐ NEUTRAL
- ☐ INSECURE
- ☐ DISCOURAGED
- ☐ DRAINED
- ☐ SAD
- ☐ SCARED
- ☐ ANGRY
- ☐ ANNOYED
- ☐ ANXIOUS
- ☐ STRESSED
- ☐ OVERWHELMED
- ☐ _____

A POSITIVE THOUGHT TO CARRY ME TO SLEEP:
_____
_____
_____

MORNING

DATE ____/____/____

TODAY'S FOCUS:
_____
_____
_____
_____

AN AFFIRMATION FOR TODAY:
_____
_____
_____

WHAT I'M GRATEFUL FOR:
_____
_____
_____
_____
_____
_____
_____
_____

WHAT I'M EXCITED ABOUT TODAY:
_____
_____
_____

HOW I'LL MAKE SPACE FOR GRATITUDE TODAY:
_____
_____
_____

EVENING

GOOD THINGS THAT HAPPENED TODAY:
_____
_____
_____
_____

THINGS I DID TO MAKE A POSITIVE DIFFERENCE TODAY:
_____
_____
_____
_____

HOW I FELT TODAY:

- ☐ HAPPY
- ☐ CONTENT
- ☐ PROUD
- ☐ HOPEFUL
- ☐ LOVING
- ☐ CONNECTED
- ☐ BALANCED
- ☐ JOYFUL
- ☐ RELAXED
- ☐ CREATIVE
- ☐ EXCITED
- ☐ _____

- ☐ NEUTRAL
- ☐ INSECURE
- ☐ DISCOURAGED
- ☐ DRAINED
- ☐ SAD
- ☐ SCARED
- ☐ ANGRY
- ☐ ANNOYED
- ☐ ANXIOUS
- ☐ STRESSED
- ☐ OVERWHELMED
- ☐ _____

A POSITIVE THOUGHT TO CARRY ME TO SLEEP:
_____
_____
_____

MORNING

DATE ___/___/___

TODAY'S FOCUS:
_____
_____
_____
_____

AN AFFIRMATION FOR TODAY:
_____
_____
_____
_____

WHAT I'M GRATEFUL FOR:
_____
_____
_____
_____
_____
_____
_____
_____

WHAT I'M EXCITED ABOUT TODAY:
_____
_____
_____

HOW I'LL MAKE SPACE FOR GRATITUDE TODAY:
_____
_____
_____

EVENING

GOOD THINGS THAT HAPPENED TODAY:
_____
_____
_____

THINGS I DID TO MAKE A POSITIVE DIFFERENCE TODAY:
_____
_____
_____

HOW I FELT TODAY:

- ☐ HAPPY
- ☐ CONTENT
- ☐ PROUD
- ☐ HOPEFUL
- ☐ LOVING
- ☐ CONNECTED
- ☐ BALANCED
- ☐ JOYFUL
- ☐ RELAXED
- ☐ CREATIVE
- ☐ EXCITED
- ☐ _____

- ☐ NEUTRAL
- ☐ INSECURE
- ☐ DISCOURAGED
- ☐ DRAINED
- ☐ SAD
- ☐ SCARED
- ☐ ANGRY
- ☐ ANNOYED
- ☐ ANXIOUS
- ☐ STRESSED
- ☐ OVERWHELMED
- ☐ _____

A POSITIVE THOUGHT TO CARRY ME TO SLEEP:
_____
_____
_____

MORNING

DATE ____/____/____

TODAY'S FOCUS:
_____
_____
_____
_____

AN AFFIRMATION FOR TODAY:
_____
_____
_____

WHAT I'M GRATEFUL FOR:
_____
_____
_____
_____
_____
_____
_____
_____
_____

WHAT I'M EXCITED ABOUT TODAY:
_____
_____
_____

HOW I'LL MAKE SPACE FOR GRATITUDE TODAY:
_____
_____
_____

EVENING

GOOD THINGS THAT HAPPENED TODAY:

___

THINGS I DID TO MAKE A POSITIVE DIFFERENCE TODAY:

___

HOW I FELT TODAY:

- ☐ HAPPY
- ☐ CONTENT
- ☐ PROUD
- ☐ HOPEFUL
- ☐ LOVING
- ☐ CONNECTED
- ☐ BALANCED
- ☐ JOYFUL
- ☐ RELAXED
- ☐ CREATIVE
- ☐ EXCITED
- ☐ _____

- ☐ NEUTRAL
- ☐ INSECURE
- ☐ DISCOURAGED
- ☐ DRAINED
- ☐ SAD
- ☐ SCARED
- ☐ ANGRY
- ☐ ANNOYED
- ☐ ANXIOUS
- ☐ STRESSED
- ☐ OVERWHELMED
- ☐ _____

A POSITIVE THOUGHT TO CARRY ME TO SLEEP:

___

MORNING

DATE ____/____/____

TODAY'S FOCUS:
_____
_____
_____
_____

AN AFFIRMATION FOR TODAY:
_____
_____
_____
_____

WHAT I'M GRATEFUL FOR:
_____
_____
_____
_____
_____
_____
_____
_____

WHAT I'M EXCITED ABOUT TODAY:
_____
_____
_____

HOW I'LL MAKE SPACE FOR GRATITUDE TODAY:
_____
_____
_____

EVENING

GOOD THINGS THAT HAPPENED TODAY:

THINGS I DID TO MAKE A POSITIVE DIFFERENCE TODAY:

HOW I FELT TODAY:

- ☐ HAPPY
- ☐ CONTENT
- ☐ PROUD
- ☐ HOPEFUL
- ☐ LOVING
- ☐ CONNECTED
- ☐ BALANCED
- ☐ JOYFUL
- ☐ RELAXED
- ☐ CREATIVE
- ☐ EXCITED
- ☐ _____

- ☐ NEUTRAL
- ☐ INSECURE
- ☐ DISCOURAGED
- ☐ DRAINED
- ☐ SAD
- ☐ SCARED
- ☐ ANGRY
- ☐ ANNOYED
- ☐ ANXIOUS
- ☐ STRESSED
- ☐ OVERWHELMED
- ☐ _____

A POSITIVE THOUGHT TO CARRY ME TO SLEEP:

MORNING

DATE ___/___/___

TODAY'S FOCUS:
_____
_____
_____
_____

AN AFFIRMATION FOR TODAY:
_____
_____
_____
_____

WHAT I'M GRATEFUL FOR:
_____
_____
_____
_____
_____
_____
_____
_____

WHAT I'M EXCITED ABOUT TODAY:
_____
_____
_____

HOW I'LL MAKE SPACE FOR GRATITUDE TODAY:
_____
_____
_____

EVENING

GOOD THINGS THAT HAPPENED TODAY:
_____
_____
_____
_____

THINGS I DID TO MAKE A POSITIVE DIFFERENCE TODAY:
_____
_____
_____
_____

HOW I FELT TODAY:

- ☐ HAPPY
- ☐ CONTENT
- ☐ PROUD
- ☐ HOPEFUL
- ☐ LOVING
- ☐ CONNECTED
- ☐ BALANCED
- ☐ JOYFUL
- ☐ RELAXED
- ☐ CREATIVE
- ☐ EXCITED
- ☐ _____

- ☐ NEUTRAL
- ☐ INSECURE
- ☐ DISCOURAGED
- ☐ DRAINED
- ☐ SAD
- ☐ SCARED
- ☐ ANGRY
- ☐ ANNOYED
- ☐ ANXIOUS
- ☐ STRESSED
- ☐ OVERWHELMED
- ☐ _____

A POSITIVE THOUGHT TO CARRY ME TO SLEEP:
_____
_____
_____

MORNING

DATE ___/___/___

TODAY'S FOCUS:

AN AFFIRMATION FOR TODAY:

WHAT I'M GRATEFUL FOR:

WHAT I'M EXCITED ABOUT TODAY:

HOW I'LL MAKE SPACE FOR GRATITUDE TODAY:

EVENING

GOOD THINGS THAT HAPPENED TODAY:

THINGS I DID TO MAKE A POSITIVE DIFFERENCE TODAY:

HOW I FELT TODAY:

- ☐ HAPPY
- ☐ CONTENT
- ☐ PROUD
- ☐ HOPEFUL
- ☐ LOVING
- ☐ CONNECTED
- ☐ BALANCED
- ☐ JOYFUL
- ☐ RELAXED
- ☐ CREATIVE
- ☐ EXCITED
- ☐ _____

- ☐ NEUTRAL
- ☐ INSECURE
- ☐ DISCOURAGED
- ☐ DRAINED
- ☐ SAD
- ☐ SCARED
- ☐ ANGRY
- ☐ ANNOYED
- ☐ ANXIOUS
- ☐ STRESSED
- ☐ OVERWHELMED
- ☐ _____

A POSITIVE THOUGHT TO CARRY ME TO SLEEP:

MORNING

DATE ___/___/___

TODAY'S FOCUS:

AN AFFIRMATION FOR TODAY:

WHAT I'M GRATEFUL FOR:

WHAT I'M EXCITED ABOUT TODAY:

HOW I'LL MAKE SPACE FOR GRATITUDE TODAY:

EVENING

GOOD THINGS THAT HAPPENED TODAY:
_____
_____
_____
_____

THINGS I DID TO MAKE A POSITIVE DIFFERENCE TODAY:
_____
_____
_____
_____

HOW I FELT TODAY:

- ☐ HAPPY
- ☐ CONTENT
- ☐ PROUD
- ☐ HOPEFUL
- ☐ LOVING
- ☐ CONNECTED
- ☐ BALANCED
- ☐ JOYFUL
- ☐ RELAXED
- ☐ CREATIVE
- ☐ EXCITED
- ☐ _____

- ☐ NEUTRAL
- ☐ INSECURE
- ☐ DISCOURAGED
- ☐ DRAINED
- ☐ SAD
- ☐ SCARED
- ☐ ANGRY
- ☐ ANNOYED
- ☐ ANXIOUS
- ☐ STRESSED
- ☐ OVERWHELMED
- ☐ _____

A POSITIVE THOUGHT TO CARRY ME TO SLEEP:
_____
_____
_____

MORNING

DATE ___/___/___

TODAY'S FOCUS:
_____
_____
_____
_____

AN AFFIRMATION FOR TODAY:
_____
_____
_____

WHAT I'M GRATEFUL FOR:
_____
_____
_____
_____
_____
_____
_____
_____

WHAT I'M EXCITED ABOUT TODAY:
_____
_____
_____

HOW I'LL MAKE SPACE FOR GRATITUDE TODAY:
_____
_____
_____

EVENING

GOOD THINGS THAT HAPPENED TODAY:
_____
_____
_____
_____

THINGS I DID TO MAKE A POSITIVE DIFFERENCE TODAY:
_____
_____
_____
_____

HOW I FELT TODAY:

- ☐ HAPPY
- ☐ CONTENT
- ☐ PROUD
- ☐ HOPEFUL
- ☐ LOVING
- ☐ CONNECTED
- ☐ BALANCED
- ☐ JOYFUL
- ☐ RELAXED
- ☐ CREATIVE
- ☐ EXCITED
- ☐ _____

- ☐ NEUTRAL
- ☐ INSECURE
- ☐ DISCOURAGED
- ☐ DRAINED
- ☐ SAD
- ☐ SCARED
- ☐ ANGRY
- ☐ ANNOYED
- ☐ ANXIOUS
- ☐ STRESSED
- ☐ OVERWHELMED
- ☐ _____

A POSITIVE THOUGHT TO CARRY ME TO SLEEP:
_____
_____
_____

MORNING

DATE ___/___/___

TODAY'S FOCUS:

AN AFFIRMATION FOR TODAY:

WHAT I'M GRATEFUL FOR:

WHAT I'M EXCITED ABOUT TODAY:

HOW I'LL MAKE SPACE FOR GRATITUDE TODAY:

EVENING

GOOD THINGS THAT HAPPENED TODAY:
_____
_____
_____
_____

THINGS I DID TO MAKE A POSITIVE DIFFERENCE TODAY:
_____
_____
_____
_____

HOW I FELT TODAY:

- ☐ HAPPY
- ☐ CONTENT
- ☐ PROUD
- ☐ HOPEFUL
- ☐ LOVING
- ☐ CONNECTED
- ☐ BALANCED
- ☐ JOYFUL
- ☐ RELAXED
- ☐ CREATIVE
- ☐ EXCITED
- ☐ _____

- ☐ NEUTRAL
- ☐ INSECURE
- ☐ DISCOURAGED
- ☐ DRAINED
- ☐ SAD
- ☐ SCARED
- ☐ ANGRY
- ☐ ANNOYED
- ☐ ANXIOUS
- ☐ STRESSED
- ☐ OVERWHELMED
- ☐ _____

A POSITIVE THOUGHT TO CARRY ME TO SLEEP:
_____
_____
_____

MORNING

DATE ____/____/____

TODAY'S FOCUS:

AN AFFIRMATION FOR TODAY:

WHAT I'M GRATEFUL FOR:

WHAT I'M EXCITED ABOUT TODAY:

HOW I'LL MAKE SPACE FOR GRATITUDE TODAY:

EVENING

GOOD THINGS THAT HAPPENED TODAY:
___
___
___
___

THINGS I DID TO MAKE A POSITIVE DIFFERENCE TODAY:
___
___
___
___

HOW I FELT TODAY:

- ☐ HAPPY
- ☐ CONTENT
- ☐ PROUD
- ☐ HOPEFUL
- ☐ LOVING
- ☐ CONNECTED
- ☐ BALANCED
- ☐ JOYFUL
- ☐ RELAXED
- ☐ CREATIVE
- ☐ EXCITED
- ☐ _____

- ☐ NEUTRAL
- ☐ INSECURE
- ☐ DISCOURAGED
- ☐ DRAINED
- ☐ SAD
- ☐ SCARED
- ☐ ANGRY
- ☐ ANNOYED
- ☐ ANXIOUS
- ☐ STRESSED
- ☐ OVERWHELMED
- ☐ _____

A POSITIVE THOUGHT TO CARRY ME TO SLEEP:
___
___
___

MORNING

DATE ___/___/___

TODAY'S FOCUS:
_____
_____
_____
_____

AN AFFIRMATION FOR TODAY:
_____
_____
_____
_____

WHAT I'M GRATEFUL FOR:
_____
_____
_____
_____
_____
_____
_____
_____
_____
_____

WHAT I'M EXCITED ABOUT TODAY:
_____
_____
_____

HOW I'LL MAKE SPACE FOR GRATITUDE TODAY:
_____
_____
_____

EVENING

GOOD THINGS THAT HAPPENED TODAY:
_____
_____
_____
_____

THINGS I DID TO MAKE A POSITIVE DIFFERENCE TODAY:
_____
_____
_____
_____

HOW I FELT TODAY:

- ☐ HAPPY
- ☐ CONTENT
- ☐ PROUD
- ☐ HOPEFUL
- ☐ LOVING
- ☐ CONNECTED
- ☐ BALANCED
- ☐ JOYFUL
- ☐ RELAXED
- ☐ CREATIVE
- ☐ EXCITED
- ☐ _____

- ☐ NEUTRAL
- ☐ INSECURE
- ☐ DISCOURAGED
- ☐ DRAINED
- ☐ SAD
- ☐ SCARED
- ☐ ANGRY
- ☐ ANNOYED
- ☐ ANXIOUS
- ☐ STRESSED
- ☐ OVERWHELMED
- ☐ _____

A POSITIVE THOUGHT TO CARRY ME TO SLEEP:
_____
_____
_____

MORNING

DATE ___/___/___

TODAY'S FOCUS:
_____
_____
_____
_____

AN AFFIRMATION FOR TODAY:
_____
_____
_____
_____

WHAT I'M GRATEFUL FOR:
_____
_____
_____
_____
_____
_____
_____
_____

WHAT I'M EXCITED ABOUT TODAY:
_____
_____
_____

HOW I'LL MAKE SPACE FOR GRATITUDE TODAY:
_____
_____
_____

EVENING

GOOD THINGS THAT HAPPENED TODAY:

THINGS I DID TO MAKE A POSITIVE DIFFERENCE TODAY:

HOW I FELT TODAY:

- [ ] HAPPY
- [ ] CONTENT
- [ ] PROUD
- [ ] HOPEFUL
- [ ] LOVING
- [ ] CONNECTED
- [ ] BALANCED
- [ ] JOYFUL
- [ ] RELAXED
- [ ] CREATIVE
- [ ] EXCITED
- [ ] _____

- [ ] NEUTRAL
- [ ] INSECURE
- [ ] DISCOURAGED
- [ ] DRAINED
- [ ] SAD
- [ ] SCARED
- [ ] ANGRY
- [ ] ANNOYED
- [ ] ANXIOUS
- [ ] STRESSED
- [ ] OVERWHELMED
- [ ] _____

A POSITIVE THOUGHT TO CARRY ME TO SLEEP:

MORNING

DATE ___/___/___

TODAY'S FOCUS:
_____
_____
_____
_____

AN AFFIRMATION FOR TODAY:
_____
_____
_____

WHAT I'M GRATEFUL FOR:
_____
_____
_____
_____
_____
_____
_____
_____
_____

WHAT I'M EXCITED ABOUT TODAY:
_____
_____
_____

HOW I'LL MAKE SPACE FOR GRATITUDE TODAY:
_____
_____
_____

EVENING

GOOD THINGS THAT HAPPENED TODAY:
_____
_____
_____
_____

THINGS I DID TO MAKE A POSITIVE DIFFERENCE TODAY:
_____
_____
_____
_____

HOW I FELT TODAY:

- ☐ HAPPY
- ☐ CONTENT
- ☐ PROUD
- ☐ HOPEFUL
- ☐ LOVING
- ☐ CONNECTED
- ☐ BALANCED
- ☐ JOYFUL
- ☐ RELAXED
- ☐ CREATIVE
- ☐ EXCITED
- ☐ _____

- ☐ NEUTRAL
- ☐ INSECURE
- ☐ DISCOURAGED
- ☐ DRAINED
- ☐ SAD
- ☐ SCARED
- ☐ ANGRY
- ☐ ANNOYED
- ☐ ANXIOUS
- ☐ STRESSED
- ☐ OVERWHELMED
- ☐ _____

A POSITIVE THOUGHT TO CARRY ME TO SLEEP:
_____
_____
_____

MORNING

DATE ___/___/___

TODAY'S FOCUS:

AN AFFIRMATION FOR TODAY:

WHAT I'M GRATEFUL FOR:

WHAT I'M EXCITED ABOUT TODAY:

HOW I'LL MAKE SPACE FOR GRATITUDE TODAY:

EVENING

GOOD THINGS THAT HAPPENED TODAY:
_____
_____
_____
_____

THINGS I DID TO MAKE A POSITIVE DIFFERENCE TODAY:
_____
_____
_____
_____

HOW I FELT TODAY:

- ☐ HAPPY
- ☐ CONTENT
- ☐ PROUD
- ☐ HOPEFUL
- ☐ LOVING
- ☐ CONNECTED
- ☐ BALANCED
- ☐ JOYFUL
- ☐ RELAXED
- ☐ CREATIVE
- ☐ EXCITED
- ☐ _____

- ☐ NEUTRAL
- ☐ INSECURE
- ☐ DISCOURAGED
- ☐ DRAINED
- ☐ SAD
- ☐ SCARED
- ☐ ANGRY
- ☐ ANNOYED
- ☐ ANXIOUS
- ☐ STRESSED
- ☐ OVERWHELMED
- ☐ _____

A POSITIVE THOUGHT TO CARRY ME TO SLEEP:
_____
_____
_____

MORNING

DATE ___/___/___

TODAY'S FOCUS:

AN AFFIRMATION FOR TODAY:

WHAT I'M GRATEFUL FOR:

WHAT I'M EXCITED ABOUT TODAY:

HOW I'LL MAKE SPACE FOR GRATITUDE TODAY:

EVENING

GOOD THINGS THAT HAPPENED TODAY:
_____
_____
_____

THINGS I DID TO MAKE A POSITIVE DIFFERENCE TODAY:
_____
_____
_____

HOW I FELT TODAY:

- ☐ HAPPY
- ☐ CONTENT
- ☐ PROUD
- ☐ HOPEFUL
- ☐ LOVING
- ☐ CONNECTED
- ☐ BALANCED
- ☐ JOYFUL
- ☐ RELAXED
- ☐ CREATIVE
- ☐ EXCITED
- ☐ _____

- ☐ NEUTRAL
- ☐ INSECURE
- ☐ DISCOURAGED
- ☐ DRAINED
- ☐ SAD
- ☐ SCARED
- ☐ ANGRY
- ☐ ANNOYED
- ☐ ANXIOUS
- ☐ STRESSED
- ☐ OVERWHELMED
- ☐ _____

_____
_____
_____
_____
_____
_____

A POSITIVE THOUGHT TO CARRY ME TO SLEEP:
_____
_____
_____

MORNING

DATE ___/___/___

TODAY'S FOCUS:

AN AFFIRMATION FOR TODAY:

WHAT I'M GRATEFUL FOR:

WHAT I'M EXCITED ABOUT TODAY:

HOW I'LL MAKE SPACE FOR GRATITUDE TODAY:

EVENING

GOOD THINGS THAT HAPPENED TODAY:
_____
_____
_____
_____

THINGS I DID TO MAKE A POSITIVE DIFFERENCE TODAY:
_____
_____
_____
_____

HOW I FELT TODAY:

- ☐ HAPPY
- ☐ CONTENT
- ☐ PROUD
- ☐ HOPEFUL
- ☐ LOVING
- ☐ CONNECTED
- ☐ BALANCED
- ☐ JOYFUL
- ☐ RELAXED
- ☐ CREATIVE
- ☐ EXCITED
- ☐ _____

- ☐ NEUTRAL
- ☐ INSECURE
- ☐ DISCOURAGED
- ☐ DRAINED
- ☐ SAD
- ☐ SCARED
- ☐ ANGRY
- ☐ ANNOYED
- ☐ ANXIOUS
- ☐ STRESSED
- ☐ OVERWHELMED
- ☐ _____

A POSITIVE THOUGHT TO CARRY ME TO SLEEP:
_____
_____
_____

MORNING

DATE ___/___/___

TODAY'S FOCUS:
_____
_____
_____
_____

AN AFFIRMATION FOR TODAY:
_____
_____
_____

WHAT I'M GRATEFUL FOR:
_____
_____
_____
_____
_____
_____
_____
_____
_____

WHAT I'M EXCITED ABOUT TODAY:
_____
_____
_____

HOW I'LL MAKE SPACE FOR GRATITUDE TODAY:
_____
_____
_____

EVENING

GOOD THINGS THAT HAPPENED TODAY:
___
___
___
___

THINGS I DID TO MAKE A POSITIVE DIFFERENCE TODAY:
___
___
___
___

HOW I FELT TODAY:

- ☐ HAPPY
- ☐ CONTENT
- ☐ PROUD
- ☐ HOPEFUL
- ☐ LOVING
- ☐ CONNECTED
- ☐ BALANCED
- ☐ JOYFUL
- ☐ RELAXED
- ☐ CREATIVE
- ☐ EXCITED
- ☐ _____

- ☐ NEUTRAL
- ☐ INSECURE
- ☐ DISCOURAGED
- ☐ DRAINED
- ☐ SAD
- ☐ SCARED
- ☐ ANGRY
- ☐ ANNOYED
- ☐ ANXIOUS
- ☐ STRESSED
- ☐ OVERWHELMED
- ☐ _____

___
___
___
___
___
___
___

A POSITIVE THOUGHT TO CARRY ME TO SLEEP:
___
___
___

MORNING

DATE ____/____/____

TODAY'S FOCUS:
_____
_____
_____
_____

AN AFFIRMATION FOR TODAY:
_____
_____
_____

WHAT I'M GRATEFUL FOR:
_____
_____
_____
_____
_____
_____
_____
_____
_____

WHAT I'M EXCITED ABOUT TODAY:
_____
_____
_____

HOW I'LL MAKE SPACE FOR GRATITUDE TODAY:
_____
_____
_____

EVENING

GOOD THINGS THAT HAPPENED TODAY:
_____
_____
_____
_____

THINGS I DID TO MAKE A POSITIVE DIFFERENCE TODAY:
_____
_____
_____
_____

HOW I FELT TODAY:

- ☐ HAPPY
- ☐ CONTENT
- ☐ PROUD
- ☐ HOPEFUL
- ☐ LOVING
- ☐ CONNECTED
- ☐ BALANCED
- ☐ JOYFUL
- ☐ RELAXED
- ☐ CREATIVE
- ☐ EXCITED
- ☐ _____

- ☐ NEUTRAL
- ☐ INSECURE
- ☐ DISCOURAGED
- ☐ DRAINED
- ☐ SAD
- ☐ SCARED
- ☐ ANGRY
- ☐ ANNOYED
- ☐ ANXIOUS
- ☐ STRESSED
- ☐ OVERWHELMED
- ☐ _____

A POSITIVE THOUGHT TO CARRY ME TO SLEEP:
_____
_____
_____

MORNING

DATE ___/___/___

TODAY'S FOCUS:
_____
_____
_____
_____

AN AFFIRMATION FOR TODAY:
_____
_____
_____
_____

WHAT I'M GRATEFUL FOR:
_____
_____
_____
_____
_____
_____
_____
_____
_____

WHAT I'M EXCITED ABOUT TODAY:
_____
_____
_____

HOW I'LL MAKE SPACE FOR GRATITUDE TODAY:
_____
_____
_____

EVENING

GOOD THINGS THAT HAPPENED TODAY:
_____
_____
_____
_____

THINGS I DID TO MAKE A POSITIVE DIFFERENCE TODAY:
_____
_____
_____
_____

HOW I FELT TODAY:

- ☐ HAPPY
- ☐ CONTENT
- ☐ PROUD
- ☐ HOPEFUL
- ☐ LOVING
- ☐ CONNECTED
- ☐ BALANCED
- ☐ JOYFUL
- ☐ RELAXED
- ☐ CREATIVE
- ☐ EXCITED
- ☐ _____

- ☐ NEUTRAL
- ☐ INSECURE
- ☐ DISCOURAGED
- ☐ DRAINED
- ☐ SAD
- ☐ SCARED
- ☐ ANGRY
- ☐ ANNOYED
- ☐ ANXIOUS
- ☐ STRESSED
- ☐ OVERWHELMED
- ☐ _____

A POSITIVE THOUGHT TO CARRY ME TO SLEEP:
_____
_____
_____

MORNING

DATE ___/___/___

TODAY'S FOCUS:

AN AFFIRMATION FOR TODAY:

WHAT I'M GRATEFUL FOR:

WHAT I'M EXCITED ABOUT TODAY:

HOW I'LL MAKE SPACE FOR GRATITUDE TODAY:

EVENING

GOOD THINGS THAT HAPPENED TODAY:
_____
_____
_____
_____

THINGS I DID TO MAKE A POSITIVE DIFFERENCE TODAY:
_____
_____
_____
_____

HOW I FELT TODAY:

- [ ] HAPPY
- [ ] CONTENT
- [ ] PROUD
- [ ] HOPEFUL
- [ ] LOVING
- [ ] CONNECTED
- [ ] BALANCED
- [ ] JOYFUL
- [ ] RELAXED
- [ ] CREATIVE
- [ ] EXCITED
- [ ] _____

- [ ] NEUTRAL
- [ ] INSECURE
- [ ] DISCOURAGED
- [ ] DRAINED
- [ ] SAD
- [ ] SCARED
- [ ] ANGRY
- [ ] ANNOYED
- [ ] ANXIOUS
- [ ] STRESSED
- [ ] OVERWHELMED
- [ ] _____

A POSITIVE THOUGHT TO CARRY ME TO SLEEP:
_____
_____
_____

MORNING

DATE ___/___/___

TODAY'S FOCUS:
_____
_____
_____
_____

AN AFFIRMATION FOR TODAY:
_____
_____
_____
_____

WHAT I'M GRATEFUL FOR:
_____
_____
_____
_____
_____
_____
_____
_____

WHAT I'M EXCITED ABOUT TODAY:
_____
_____
_____

HOW I'LL MAKE SPACE FOR GRATITUDE TODAY:
_____
_____
_____

EVENING

GOOD THINGS THAT HAPPENED TODAY:
_____
_____
_____
_____

THINGS I DID TO MAKE A POSITIVE DIFFERENCE TODAY:
_____
_____
_____
_____

HOW I FELT TODAY:

- [ ] HAPPY
- [ ] CONTENT
- [ ] PROUD
- [ ] HOPEFUL
- [ ] LOVING
- [ ] CONNECTED
- [ ] BALANCED
- [ ] JOYFUL
- [ ] RELAXED
- [ ] CREATIVE
- [ ] EXCITED
- [ ] _____

- [ ] NEUTRAL
- [ ] INSECURE
- [ ] DISCOURAGED
- [ ] DRAINED
- [ ] SAD
- [ ] SCARED
- [ ] ANGRY
- [ ] ANNOYED
- [ ] ANXIOUS
- [ ] STRESSED
- [ ] OVERWHELMED
- [ ] _____

_____
_____
_____
_____
_____
_____

A POSITIVE THOUGHT TO CARRY ME TO SLEEP:
_____
_____
_____

MORNING

DATE ___/___/___

TODAY'S FOCUS:
_____
_____
_____
_____

AN AFFIRMATION FOR TODAY:
_____
_____
_____
_____

WHAT I'M GRATEFUL FOR:
_____
_____
_____
_____
_____
_____
_____
_____
_____

WHAT I'M EXCITED ABOUT TODAY:
_____
_____
_____

HOW I'LL MAKE SPACE FOR GRATITUDE TODAY:
_____
_____
_____

EVENING

GOOD THINGS THAT HAPPENED TODAY:
_____
_____
_____
_____

THINGS I DID TO MAKE A POSITIVE DIFFERENCE TODAY:
_____
_____
_____
_____

HOW I FELT TODAY:

- ☐ HAPPY
- ☐ CONTENT
- ☐ PROUD
- ☐ HOPEFUL
- ☐ LOVING
- ☐ CONNECTED
- ☐ BALANCED
- ☐ JOYFUL
- ☐ RELAXED
- ☐ CREATIVE
- ☐ EXCITED
- ☐ _____

- ☐ NEUTRAL
- ☐ INSECURE
- ☐ DISCOURAGED
- ☐ DRAINED
- ☐ SAD
- ☐ SCARED
- ☐ ANGRY
- ☐ ANNOYED
- ☐ ANXIOUS
- ☐ STRESSED
- ☐ OVERWHELMED
- ☐ _____

A POSITIVE THOUGHT TO CARRY ME TO SLEEP:
_____
_____
_____

MORNING

DATE ___/___/___

TODAY'S FOCUS:
_____
_____
_____
_____

AN AFFIRMATION FOR TODAY:
_____
_____
_____
_____

WHAT I'M GRATEFUL FOR:
_____
_____
_____
_____
_____
_____
_____
_____

WHAT I'M EXCITED ABOUT TODAY:
_____
_____

HOW I'LL MAKE SPACE FOR GRATITUDE TODAY:
_____
_____
_____

EVENING

GOOD THINGS THAT HAPPENED TODAY:
_____
_____
_____
_____

THINGS I DID TO MAKE A POSITIVE DIFFERENCE TODAY:
_____
_____
_____
_____

HOW I FELT TODAY:

- ☐ HAPPY
- ☐ CONTENT
- ☐ PROUD
- ☐ HOPEFUL
- ☐ LOVING
- ☐ CONNECTED
- ☐ BALANCED
- ☐ JOYFUL
- ☐ RELAXED
- ☐ CREATIVE
- ☐ EXCITED
- ☐ _____

- ☐ NEUTRAL
- ☐ INSECURE
- ☐ DISCOURAGED
- ☐ DRAINED
- ☐ SAD
- ☐ SCARED
- ☐ ANGRY
- ☐ ANNOYED
- ☐ ANXIOUS
- ☐ STRESSED
- ☐ OVERWHELMED
- ☐ _____

A POSITIVE THOUGHT TO CARRY ME TO SLEEP:
_____
_____
_____

MORNING

DATE ___/___/___

TODAY'S FOCUS:
_____
_____
_____
_____

AN AFFIRMATION FOR TODAY:
_____
_____
_____
_____

WHAT I'M GRATEFUL FOR:
_____
_____
_____
_____
_____
_____
_____
_____
_____

WHAT I'M EXCITED ABOUT TODAY:
_____
_____
_____

HOW I'LL MAKE SPACE FOR GRATITUDE TODAY:
_____
_____
_____

EVENING

GOOD THINGS THAT HAPPENED TODAY:
_____
_____
_____
_____

THINGS I DID TO MAKE A POSITIVE DIFFERENCE TODAY:
_____
_____
_____
_____

HOW I FELT TODAY:

- ☐ HAPPY
- ☐ CONTENT
- ☐ PROUD
- ☐ HOPEFUL
- ☐ LOVING
- ☐ CONNECTED
- ☐ BALANCED
- ☐ JOYFUL
- ☐ RELAXED
- ☐ CREATIVE
- ☐ EXCITED
- ☐ _____

- ☐ NEUTRAL
- ☐ INSECURE
- ☐ DISCOURAGED
- ☐ DRAINED
- ☐ SAD
- ☐ SCARED
- ☐ ANGRY
- ☐ ANNOYED
- ☐ ANXIOUS
- ☐ STRESSED
- ☐ OVERWHELMED
- ☐ _____

A POSITIVE THOUGHT TO CARRY ME TO SLEEP:
_____
_____
_____

MORNING

DATE ___/___/___

TODAY'S FOCUS:

AN AFFIRMATION FOR TODAY:

WHAT I'M GRATEFUL FOR:

WHAT I'M EXCITED ABOUT TODAY:

HOW I'LL MAKE SPACE FOR GRATITUDE TODAY:

EVENING

GOOD THINGS THAT HAPPENED TODAY:
_____
_____
_____
_____

THINGS I DID TO MAKE A POSITIVE DIFFERENCE TODAY:
_____
_____
_____
_____

HOW I FELT TODAY:

- ☐ HAPPY
- ☐ CONTENT
- ☐ PROUD
- ☐ HOPEFUL
- ☐ LOVING
- ☐ CONNECTED
- ☐ BALANCED
- ☐ JOYFUL
- ☐ RELAXED
- ☐ CREATIVE
- ☐ EXCITED
- ☐ _____

- ☐ NEUTRAL
- ☐ INSECURE
- ☐ DISCOURAGED
- ☐ DRAINED
- ☐ SAD
- ☐ SCARED
- ☐ ANGRY
- ☐ ANNOYED
- ☐ ANXIOUS
- ☐ STRESSED
- ☐ OVERWHELMED
- ☐ _____

A POSITIVE THOUGHT TO CARRY ME TO SLEEP:
_____
_____
_____

MORNING

DATE ___/___/___

TODAY'S FOCUS:
_____
_____
_____
_____

AN AFFIRMATION FOR TODAY:
_____
_____
_____

WHAT I'M GRATEFUL FOR:
_____
_____
_____
_____
_____
_____
_____
_____

WHAT I'M EXCITED ABOUT TODAY:
_____
_____

HOW I'LL MAKE SPACE FOR GRATITUDE TODAY:
_____
_____
_____

EVENING

GOOD THINGS THAT HAPPENED TODAY:
___

THINGS I DID TO MAKE A POSITIVE DIFFERENCE TODAY:
___

HOW I FELT TODAY:

- ☐ HAPPY
- ☐ CONTENT
- ☐ PROUD
- ☐ HOPEFUL
- ☐ LOVING
- ☐ CONNECTED
- ☐ BALANCED
- ☐ JOYFUL
- ☐ RELAXED
- ☐ CREATIVE
- ☐ EXCITED
- ☐ _____

- ☐ NEUTRAL
- ☐ INSECURE
- ☐ DISCOURAGED
- ☐ DRAINED
- ☐ SAD
- ☐ SCARED
- ☐ ANGRY
- ☐ ANNOYED
- ☐ ANXIOUS
- ☐ STRESSED
- ☐ OVERWHELMED
- ☐ _____

A POSITIVE THOUGHT TO CARRY ME TO SLEEP:
___

MORNING

DATE ___/___/___

TODAY'S FOCUS:

AN AFFIRMATION FOR TODAY:

WHAT I'M GRATEFUL FOR:

WHAT I'M EXCITED ABOUT TODAY:

HOW I'LL MAKE SPACE FOR GRATITUDE TODAY:

EVENING

GOOD THINGS THAT HAPPENED TODAY:
_____
_____
_____
_____

THINGS I DID TO MAKE A POSITIVE DIFFERENCE TODAY:
_____
_____
_____
_____

HOW I FELT TODAY:

- ☐ HAPPY
- ☐ CONTENT
- ☐ PROUD
- ☐ HOPEFUL
- ☐ LOVING
- ☐ CONNECTED
- ☐ BALANCED
- ☐ JOYFUL
- ☐ RELAXED
- ☐ CREATIVE
- ☐ EXCITED
- ☐ _____

- ☐ NEUTRAL
- ☐ INSECURE
- ☐ DISCOURAGED
- ☐ DRAINED
- ☐ SAD
- ☐ SCARED
- ☐ ANGRY
- ☐ ANNOYED
- ☐ ANXIOUS
- ☐ STRESSED
- ☐ OVERWHELMED
- ☐ _____

A POSITIVE THOUGHT TO CARRY ME TO SLEEP:
_____
_____
_____

MORNING

DATE ___/___/___

TODAY'S FOCUS:
_____
_____
_____
_____

AN AFFIRMATION FOR TODAY:
_____
_____
_____
_____

WHAT I'M GRATEFUL FOR:
_____
_____
_____
_____
_____
_____
_____
_____
_____

WHAT I'M EXCITED ABOUT TODAY:
_____
_____
_____

HOW I'LL MAKE SPACE FOR GRATITUDE TODAY:
_____
_____
_____

EVENING

GOOD THINGS THAT HAPPENED TODAY:

THINGS I DID TO MAKE A POSITIVE DIFFERENCE TODAY:

HOW I FELT TODAY:

- [ ] HAPPY
- [ ] CONTENT
- [ ] PROUD
- [ ] HOPEFUL
- [ ] LOVING
- [ ] CONNECTED
- [ ] BALANCED
- [ ] JOYFUL
- [ ] RELAXED
- [ ] CREATIVE
- [ ] EXCITED
- [ ] _____

- [ ] NEUTRAL
- [ ] INSECURE
- [ ] DISCOURAGED
- [ ] DRAINED
- [ ] SAD
- [ ] SCARED
- [ ] ANGRY
- [ ] ANNOYED
- [ ] ANXIOUS
- [ ] STRESSED
- [ ] OVERWHELMED
- [ ] _____

A POSITIVE THOUGHT TO CARRY ME TO SLEEP:

MORNING

DATE ____/____/____

TODAY'S FOCUS:
_____
_____
_____
_____

AN AFFIRMATION FOR TODAY:
_____
_____
_____
_____

WHAT I'M GRATEFUL FOR:
_____
_____
_____
_____
_____
_____
_____
_____
_____

WHAT I'M EXCITED ABOUT TODAY:
_____
_____
_____

HOW I'LL MAKE SPACE FOR GRATITUDE TODAY:
_____
_____
_____

EVENING

GOOD THINGS THAT HAPPENED TODAY:
_____
_____
_____
_____

THINGS I DID TO MAKE A POSITIVE DIFFERENCE TODAY:
_____
_____
_____
_____

HOW I FELT TODAY:

- ☐ HAPPY
- ☐ CONTENT
- ☐ PROUD
- ☐ HOPEFUL
- ☐ LOVING
- ☐ CONNECTED
- ☐ BALANCED
- ☐ JOYFUL
- ☐ RELAXED
- ☐ CREATIVE
- ☐ EXCITED
- ☐ _____

- ☐ NEUTRAL
- ☐ INSECURE
- ☐ DISCOURAGED
- ☐ DRAINED
- ☐ SAD
- ☐ SCARED
- ☐ ANGRY
- ☐ ANNOYED
- ☐ ANXIOUS
- ☐ STRESSED
- ☐ OVERWHELMED
- ☐ _____

A POSITIVE THOUGHT TO CARRY ME TO SLEEP:
_____
_____
_____

MORNING

DATE ___/___/___

TODAY'S FOCUS:
_____
_____
_____
_____

AN AFFIRMATION FOR TODAY:
_____
_____
_____
_____

WHAT I'M GRATEFUL FOR:
_____
_____
_____
_____
_____
_____
_____
_____
_____

WHAT I'M EXCITED ABOUT TODAY:
_____
_____
_____

HOW I'LL MAKE SPACE FOR GRATITUDE TODAY:
_____
_____
_____

EVENING

GOOD THINGS THAT HAPPENED TODAY:
_____
_____
_____
_____

THINGS I DID TO MAKE A POSITIVE DIFFERENCE TODAY:
_____
_____
_____
_____

HOW I FELT TODAY:

- ☐ HAPPY
- ☐ CONTENT
- ☐ PROUD
- ☐ HOPEFUL
- ☐ LOVING
- ☐ CONNECTED
- ☐ BALANCED
- ☐ JOYFUL
- ☐ RELAXED
- ☐ CREATIVE
- ☐ EXCITED
- ☐ _____

- ☐ NEUTRAL
- ☐ INSECURE
- ☐ DISCOURAGED
- ☐ DRAINED
- ☐ SAD
- ☐ SCARED
- ☐ ANGRY
- ☐ ANNOYED
- ☐ ANXIOUS
- ☐ STRESSED
- ☐ OVERWHELMED
- ☐ _____

A POSITIVE THOUGHT TO CARRY ME TO SLEEP:
_____
_____
_____

MORNING

DATE ___/___/___

TODAY'S FOCUS:
_____
_____
_____
_____

AN AFFIRMATION FOR TODAY:
_____
_____
_____
_____

WHAT I'M GRATEFUL FOR:
_____
_____
_____
_____
_____
_____
_____
_____

WHAT I'M EXCITED ABOUT TODAY:
_____
_____
_____

HOW I'LL MAKE SPACE FOR GRATITUDE TODAY:
_____
_____
_____

EVENING

GOOD THINGS THAT HAPPENED TODAY:
_____
_____
_____
_____

THINGS I DID TO MAKE A POSITIVE DIFFERENCE TODAY:
_____
_____
_____
_____

HOW I FELT TODAY:

- ☐ HAPPY
- ☐ CONTENT
- ☐ PROUD
- ☐ HOPEFUL
- ☐ LOVING
- ☐ CONNECTED
- ☐ BALANCED
- ☐ JOYFUL
- ☐ RELAXED
- ☐ CREATIVE
- ☐ EXCITED
- ☐ _____

- ☐ NEUTRAL
- ☐ INSECURE
- ☐ DISCOURAGED
- ☐ DRAINED
- ☐ SAD
- ☐ SCARED
- ☐ ANGRY
- ☐ ANNOYED
- ☐ ANXIOUS
- ☐ STRESSED
- ☐ OVERWHELMED
- ☐ _____

A POSITIVE THOUGHT TO CARRY ME TO SLEEP:
_____
_____
_____

MORNING

DATE ___/___/___

TODAY'S FOCUS:
_____
_____
_____
_____

AN AFFIRMATION FOR TODAY:
_____
_____
_____

WHAT I'M GRATEFUL FOR:
_____
_____
_____
_____
_____
_____
_____
_____
_____

WHAT I'M EXCITED ABOUT TODAY:
_____
_____
_____

HOW I'LL MAKE SPACE FOR GRATITUDE TODAY:
_____
_____
_____

EVENING

GOOD THINGS THAT HAPPENED TODAY:
_____
_____
_____
_____

THINGS I DID TO MAKE A POSITIVE DIFFERENCE TODAY:
_____
_____
_____
_____

HOW I FELT TODAY:

- [ ] HAPPY
- [ ] CONTENT
- [ ] PROUD
- [ ] HOPEFUL
- [ ] LOVING
- [ ] CONNECTED
- [ ] BALANCED
- [ ] JOYFUL
- [ ] RELAXED
- [ ] CREATIVE
- [ ] EXCITED
- [ ] _____

- [ ] NEUTRAL
- [ ] INSECURE
- [ ] DISCOURAGED
- [ ] DRAINED
- [ ] SAD
- [ ] SCARED
- [ ] ANGRY
- [ ] ANNOYED
- [ ] ANXIOUS
- [ ] STRESSED
- [ ] OVERWHELMED
- [ ] _____

A POSITIVE THOUGHT TO CARRY ME TO SLEEP:
_____
_____
_____

MORNING

DATE ___/___/___

TODAY'S FOCUS:
_____
_____
_____
_____

AN AFFIRMATION FOR TODAY:
_____
_____
_____

WHAT I'M GRATEFUL FOR:
_____
_____
_____
_____
_____
_____
_____
_____

WHAT I'M EXCITED ABOUT TODAY:
_____
_____
_____

HOW I'LL MAKE SPACE FOR GRATITUDE TODAY:
_____
_____
_____

EVENING

GOOD THINGS THAT HAPPENED TODAY:
_____
_____
_____
_____

THINGS I DID TO MAKE A POSITIVE DIFFERENCE TODAY:
_____
_____
_____
_____

HOW I FELT TODAY:

- ☐ HAPPY
- ☐ CONTENT
- ☐ PROUD
- ☐ HOPEFUL
- ☐ LOVING
- ☐ CONNECTED
- ☐ BALANCED
- ☐ JOYFUL
- ☐ RELAXED
- ☐ CREATIVE
- ☐ EXCITED
- ☐ _____

- ☐ NEUTRAL
- ☐ INSECURE
- ☐ DISCOURAGED
- ☐ DRAINED
- ☐ SAD
- ☐ SCARED
- ☐ ANGRY
- ☐ ANNOYED
- ☐ ANXIOUS
- ☐ STRESSED
- ☐ OVERWHELMED
- ☐ _____

A POSITIVE THOUGHT TO CARRY ME TO SLEEP:
_____
_____
_____

MORNING

DATE ___/___/___

TODAY'S FOCUS:

AN AFFIRMATION FOR TODAY:

WHAT I'M GRATEFUL FOR:

WHAT I'M EXCITED ABOUT TODAY:

HOW I'LL MAKE SPACE FOR GRATITUDE TODAY:

EVENING

GOOD THINGS THAT HAPPENED TODAY:
_____
_____
_____
_____

THINGS I DID TO MAKE A POSITIVE DIFFERENCE TODAY:
_____
_____
_____
_____

HOW I FELT TODAY:

- ☐ HAPPY
- ☐ CONTENT
- ☐ PROUD
- ☐ HOPEFUL
- ☐ LOVING
- ☐ CONNECTED
- ☐ BALANCED
- ☐ JOYFUL
- ☐ RELAXED
- ☐ CREATIVE
- ☐ EXCITED
- ☐ _____

- ☐ NEUTRAL
- ☐ INSECURE
- ☐ DISCOURAGED
- ☐ DRAINED
- ☐ SAD
- ☐ SCARED
- ☐ ANGRY
- ☐ ANNOYED
- ☐ ANXIOUS
- ☐ STRESSED
- ☐ OVERWHELMED
- ☐ _____

A POSITIVE THOUGHT TO CARRY ME TO SLEEP:
_____
_____
_____

MORNING

DATE ___/___/___

TODAY'S FOCUS:
_____
_____
_____
_____

AN AFFIRMATION FOR TODAY:
_____
_____
_____

WHAT I'M GRATEFUL FOR:
_____
_____
_____
_____
_____
_____
_____
_____

WHAT I'M EXCITED ABOUT TODAY:
_____
_____
_____

HOW I'LL MAKE SPACE FOR GRATITUDE TODAY:
_____
_____

EVENING

GOOD THINGS THAT HAPPENED TODAY:
_____
_____
_____
_____

THINGS I DID TO MAKE A POSITIVE DIFFERENCE TODAY:
_____
_____
_____
_____

HOW I FELT TODAY:

- ☐ HAPPY
- ☐ CONTENT
- ☐ PROUD
- ☐ HOPEFUL
- ☐ LOVING
- ☐ CONNECTED
- ☐ BALANCED
- ☐ JOYFUL
- ☐ RELAXED
- ☐ CREATIVE
- ☐ EXCITED
- ☐ _____

- ☐ NEUTRAL
- ☐ INSECURE
- ☐ DISCOURAGED
- ☐ DRAINED
- ☐ SAD
- ☐ SCARED
- ☐ ANGRY
- ☐ ANNOYED
- ☐ ANXIOUS
- ☐ STRESSED
- ☐ OVERWHELMED
- ☐ _____

A POSITIVE THOUGHT TO CARRY ME TO SLEEP:
_____
_____
_____

MORNING

DATE ___/___/___

TODAY'S FOCUS:
_____
_____
_____
_____

AN AFFIRMATION FOR TODAY:
_____
_____
_____

WHAT I'M GRATEFUL FOR:
_____
_____
_____
_____
_____
_____
_____
_____

WHAT I'M EXCITED ABOUT TODAY:
_____
_____
_____

HOW I'LL MAKE SPACE FOR GRATITUDE TODAY:
_____
_____
_____

EVENING

GOOD THINGS THAT HAPPENED TODAY:
_____
_____
_____
_____

THINGS I DID TO MAKE A POSITIVE DIFFERENCE TODAY:
_____
_____
_____
_____

HOW I FELT TODAY:

- [ ] HAPPY
- [ ] CONTENT
- [ ] PROUD
- [ ] HOPEFUL
- [ ] LOVING
- [ ] CONNECTED
- [ ] BALANCED
- [ ] JOYFUL
- [ ] RELAXED
- [ ] CREATIVE
- [ ] EXCITED
- [ ] _____

- [ ] NEUTRAL
- [ ] INSECURE
- [ ] DISCOURAGED
- [ ] DRAINED
- [ ] SAD
- [ ] SCARED
- [ ] ANGRY
- [ ] ANNOYED
- [ ] ANXIOUS
- [ ] STRESSED
- [ ] OVERWHELMED
- [ ] _____

A POSITIVE THOUGHT TO CARRY ME TO SLEEP:
_____
_____
_____

MORNING

DATE ___/___/___

TODAY'S FOCUS:

AN AFFIRMATION FOR TODAY:

WHAT I'M GRATEFUL FOR:

WHAT I'M EXCITED ABOUT TODAY:

HOW I'LL MAKE SPACE FOR GRATITUDE TODAY:

EVENING

GOOD THINGS THAT HAPPENED TODAY:
_____
_____
_____
_____

THINGS I DID TO MAKE A POSITIVE DIFFERENCE TODAY:
_____
_____
_____
_____

HOW I FELT TODAY:

- ☐ HAPPY
- ☐ CONTENT
- ☐ PROUD
- ☐ HOPEFUL
- ☐ LOVING
- ☐ CONNECTED
- ☐ BALANCED
- ☐ JOYFUL
- ☐ RELAXED
- ☐ CREATIVE
- ☐ EXCITED
- ☐ _____

- ☐ NEUTRAL
- ☐ INSECURE
- ☐ DISCOURAGED
- ☐ DRAINED
- ☐ SAD
- ☐ SCARED
- ☐ ANGRY
- ☐ ANNOYED
- ☐ ANXIOUS
- ☐ STRESSED
- ☐ OVERWHELMED
- ☐ _____

_____
_____
_____
_____
_____
_____

A POSITIVE THOUGHT TO CARRY ME TO SLEEP:
_____
_____
_____

MORNING

DATE ___/___/___

TODAY'S FOCUS:

AN AFFIRMATION FOR TODAY:

WHAT I'M GRATEFUL FOR:

WHAT I'M EXCITED ABOUT TODAY:

HOW I'LL MAKE SPACE FOR GRATITUDE TODAY:

EVENING

GOOD THINGS THAT HAPPENED TODAY:

_____
_____
_____
_____

THINGS I DID TO MAKE A POSITIVE DIFFERENCE TODAY:

_____
_____
_____
_____

HOW I FELT TODAY:

- ☐ HAPPY
- ☐ CONTENT
- ☐ PROUD
- ☐ HOPEFUL
- ☐ LOVING
- ☐ CONNECTED
- ☐ BALANCED
- ☐ JOYFUL
- ☐ RELAXED
- ☐ CREATIVE
- ☐ EXCITED
- ☐ _____

- ☐ NEUTRAL
- ☐ INSECURE
- ☐ DISCOURAGED
- ☐ DRAINED
- ☐ SAD
- ☐ SCARED
- ☐ ANGRY
- ☐ ANNOYED
- ☐ ANXIOUS
- ☐ STRESSED
- ☐ OVERWHELMED
- ☐ _____

A POSITIVE THOUGHT TO CARRY ME TO SLEEP:

_____
_____
_____

MORNING

DATE ___ / ___ / ___

TODAY'S FOCUS:
_____
_____
_____
_____

AN AFFIRMATION FOR TODAY:
_____
_____
_____
_____

WHAT I'M GRATEFUL FOR:
_____
_____
_____
_____
_____
_____
_____
_____
_____

WHAT I'M EXCITED ABOUT TODAY:
_____
_____
_____

HOW I'LL MAKE SPACE FOR GRATITUDE TODAY:
_____
_____
_____

EVENING

GOOD THINGS THAT HAPPENED TODAY:
_____
_____
_____
_____

THINGS I DID TO MAKE A POSITIVE DIFFERENCE TODAY:
_____
_____
_____
_____

HOW I FELT TODAY:

- ☐ HAPPY
- ☐ CONTENT
- ☐ PROUD
- ☐ HOPEFUL
- ☐ LOVING
- ☐ CONNECTED
- ☐ BALANCED
- ☐ JOYFUL
- ☐ RELAXED
- ☐ CREATIVE
- ☐ EXCITED
- ☐ _____

- ☐ NEUTRAL
- ☐ INSECURE
- ☐ DISCOURAGED
- ☐ DRAINED
- ☐ SAD
- ☐ SCARED
- ☐ ANGRY
- ☐ ANNOYED
- ☐ ANXIOUS
- ☐ STRESSED
- ☐ OVERWHELMED
- ☐ _____

A POSITIVE THOUGHT TO CARRY ME TO SLEEP:
_____
_____

MORNING

DATE ___/___/___

TODAY'S FOCUS:
_____
_____
_____
_____

AN AFFIRMATION FOR TODAY:
_____
_____
_____
_____

WHAT I'M GRATEFUL FOR:
_____
_____
_____
_____
_____
_____
_____
_____
_____

WHAT I'M EXCITED ABOUT TODAY:
_____
_____
_____

HOW I'LL MAKE SPACE FOR GRATITUDE TODAY:
_____
_____
_____

EVENING

GOOD THINGS THAT HAPPENED TODAY:
_____
_____
_____
_____

THINGS I DID TO MAKE A POSITIVE DIFFERENCE TODAY:
_____
_____
_____
_____

HOW I FELT TODAY:

- ☐ HAPPY
- ☐ CONTENT
- ☐ PROUD
- ☐ HOPEFUL
- ☐ LOVING
- ☐ CONNECTED
- ☐ BALANCED
- ☐ JOYFUL
- ☐ RELAXED
- ☐ CREATIVE
- ☐ EXCITED
- ☐ _____

- ☐ NEUTRAL
- ☐ INSECURE
- ☐ DISCOURAGED
- ☐ DRAINED
- ☐ SAD
- ☐ SCARED
- ☐ ANGRY
- ☐ ANNOYED
- ☐ ANXIOUS
- ☐ STRESSED
- ☐ OVERWHELMED
- ☐ _____

A POSITIVE THOUGHT TO CARRY ME TO SLEEP:
_____
_____
_____

INSIGHTS
A Mandala Journal

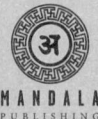

www.mandalaearth.com

Copyright © 2018 Mandala Publishing. All rights reserved.
This edition published by Mandala Publishing, San Rafael, California, in 2020.
Original edition first published by Mandala Publishing, San Rafael, California, in 2018.

MANUFACTURED IN CHINA
10 9 8 7 6 5 4 3 2